# Jump Start with ● WebLinks

## A Guidebook for Nutrition, 98/99

### Eileen L. Daniel, Ph.D.
State University of New York, College at Brockport

## Morton Publishing Company
925 W. Kenyon Avenue, Unit 12
Englewood, CO 80110

http://www.morton-pub.com

Professor Daniel, a registered dietitian, is an associate professor in the Department of Health Science at the State University of New York, College at Brockport. She received a B.S. in Nutrition and Dietetics from the Rochester Institute of Technology, a master's degree in Community Health Education from SUNY College at Brockport, and a doctorate in Health Education from the University of Oregon. A member of the Eta Sigma Gamma National Health Honor Society, the American Dietetics Association, the New York State Dietetics Association, and other professional and community organizations, she is the author or co-author of over thirty articles on issues of health, nutrition, and health education, which have appeared in such professional journals as the *Journal of Health Education* and the *Journal of College Student Development*. She is the editor of *Taking Sides: Clashing Views on Controversial Issues in Health and Society* (DPG, 1998).

---

**Credits:**
Interior Design: Joanne R. Saliger
Cover Design: Bob Schram, Bookends
Typography: Ash Street Typecrafters, Inc.
WebLinks Logo: Laura Patchkofsky

**For Morton Publishing Company:**
Douglas N. Morton, President and Publisher
Mimi Egan, Publisher, Series Publishing
Maureen Owen, Senior Editor, Series Publishing


**JumpStart with WebLinks: A Guidebook for Nutrition, 98/99**

Copyright © 1998, Morton Publishing Company
925 W. Kenyon Avenue, Unit 12
Englewood, Colorado 80110

ISBN: 0-89582-409-4

5   4   3   2   1

Printed in the United States of America

# WebAdvisory Board

Members of the WebAdvisory Board provide feedback on topics and World Wide Web sites and generally advise the guidebook's author/editor and the publishing staff. Sites have been reviewed for content, appropriateness, accessibility, and currency, and critical input is solicited from the Board for each revision of *JumpStart with WebLinks*. WebAdvisory Board Members are drawn from colleges and universities throughout the United States and Canada. They are academics with a variety of specialties and teaching experiences.

Because Morton Publishing Company also values the perspective students bring to course material, student advisors are instrumental in shaping *JumpStart with WebLinks*.

Paul Addis
University of Minnesota

Jenni Beary
University of New Mexico

Allan Davison
Simon Fraser University

Juliet Getty
University of North Texas

Amy Goodall
Student Advisor
Western Oregon University

Charlene Hamilton
University of Delaware

Barbara Hopkins
Georgia State University

Ken Kambis
College of William and Mary

Elaine Long
Boise State University

Pat Luoto
Framingham State College

Kyran J. Owen-Mankovich
Student Advisor
University of Colorado-Boulder

Millicent Owens
College of the Sequoias

Carole Sloan
Henry Ford Community College

Peggy Tinsley
Southwest Missouri
   State University

# A Note from the Publisher

## Welcome to *JumpStart with WebLinks!*

Alert and adventurous readers are important to us in keeping our guidebook up-to-date and accurate. So if you happen upon a great site, discover a location with compelling resources, find an error (it happens), or want to suggest topics for inclusion, we'd appreciate hearing from you. Just drop us a line at:

> **Morton Publishing Company**
> ⊠ 925 W. Kenyon Avenue, Unit 12
> Englewood, CO  80110
>
> e e-mail:  morton@morton-pub.com
>
> ⬛ via the Web:  http://www. morton-pub.com

### How Does a WWW Site Become a WebLink?

A World Wide Web site becomes a WebLink after it has been put through a screening process by our academic author/editor, the student advisor, and the publishing staff. To become a WebLink, a WWW site must be:

- *accessible*—all addresses/URLs (Uniform Resource Locators) have been checked and fully verified. You just enter the address directly into the Location bar on your screen and you get to the site;

- *appropriate*—the sites are reviewed for content, and contain credible information.

### You Can Count on Us

Our mission in developing this guidebook is simple: to make the resources of the World Wide Web accessible and usable within a course specific context. The exponential growth of information on the WWW is a blessing and a curse. Vast repositories of valuable information are within reach. However, finding just what you need among the tons of irrelevant information can be all but impossible. *JumpStart with WebLinks,* by rating and filtering WWW sites, can help you turn terabytes of digital noise into information you can use in your courses. You can count on our commitment to deliver a high-quality guidebook at a reasonable price on topics that are important to you. And we sincerely welcome your feedback!

# Table of Contents

# How to Use this Book

This book contains 34 topics in contemporary nutrition. For each topic, you will find:

**a topic introduction.** The topic introduction will provide you with basic information on the topic and, in some instances, current statistics. Within the topic introduction, print sources of information are cited in parentheses, in the event that you would like to check out an original print source more completely. Each topic introduction concludes with:

**questions for critical thinking.** These are a mix of content-related and personal assessment questions. Use them as study guides, or to fuel your research on the Web. After the questions for critical thinking, you will find a list of annotated World Wide Web sites. This feature is called:

**WebLinks.** These are WWWeb sites that relate to the topic. You will see that each Web site has been assigned a descriptive heading and a number. For each site, the exact address, or Universal Resource Locator, is provided. (Here is an example of a site's descriptive heading with its assigned number: *The Vegetarian Resource Group, No. 140*. Its address or URL is: http://www.vrg.org.) Next you will see that there are two pages per topic called:

**Making Your Own Connections.** Use these pages to make note of sites you have visited. You could record your reactions to a site, or briefly note what information you found there. This way, you can bring to class or turn in to your professor a paper record of where you have been on the Web. Or use these pages to jot down what you would like to discuss in class about a site.

## Accessing a Web Site

You will need to be at a computer that is hooked to the Internet and has a graphical browser—that is the software that allows you to access the World Wide Web. (The most popular browsers are Netscape and Mosaic). Once you have opened Netscape or Mosaic, delete the address that appears in the Location bar. Then, *carefully* type the address or URL of the Web site into the Location bar (or Go To bar) on the screen and press the Enter key.

The screen may look something like this after you have typed in the address:

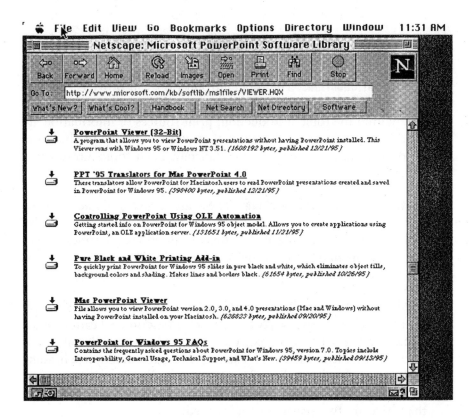

There are many ways to visit cyberspace, and this book is designed to be a guide to academically appropriate Web sites. Use it for research for class assignments, or to follow your own interests.

## Updates to WebLinks (http://www.morton-pub.com/updates/updates.stml)

Using the Web as an academic resource is not without its frustrations and limitations! You type the complete address for a site into the Location bar and, to your dismay, you don't get the results you are expecting. The site doesn't load, or it no longer exists, or the site has moved to a new location but no forwarding address or link has been provided. It is like going to the library to check out a book that is supposed to be on reserve for your course only to discover that it is not there.

At our Morton Publishing Company Web site, we are developing a section dedicated to keeping you updated about the Web addresses listed in our books that we discover are no longer operational for one reason or another. Although we carefully verify all Web addresses just prior to a book's publication, and although the publishing staff and academic editor select reputable, stable sites that will in all likelihood exist for some time, Web addresses can change or go out of service. It's the nature of the technology. Should you be unable to access a site and think that the problem is not with the server, time of day, how you entered the address, etc., go to the *Updates to WebLinks* section of the Morton Web site (http://www.morton-pub.com/updates/updates.stml), scroll down to the title of the book you are using, and click on the *Update!* icon to see if we have recommended a replacement site or a new address. (See p. x for a copy of the Morton home page.)

## The Appendices at the Back of the Book

There are several additional features of *JumpStart with WebLinks: A Guidebook for Nutrition, 98/99,* which you will find at the back of the book. Each appendix is designed to support your course work in nutrition and to maximize your time online.

Appendix A explains how to read **the new food labels**. Appendix B has **tips for citing Web sites**. The pages in Appendix C, entitled "**Your Personal Address Book**," can be used for keeping track of sites you come across when you are not online—for example, when you are reading a newspaper or magazine, watching television, or talking with a friend who recommends a site to you. Use these pages to make note of the addresses you hear about or read about when you are not at your computer, and then check them out when you are back online.

**The Web Site Evaluation Form** in Appendix D can be used in any of a number of ways: use it to evaluate Web sites that are assigned for extra credit or as a tool to assist you if you are preparing a research assignment. Even if your instructor does not require you to use the Web Site Evaluation Form, we encourage you to make photocopies of it and use it to direct your work on the Web. The questions in the form will help you to apply critical thinking skill to online sources of information.

## Index

All the Web sites that appear in *JumpStart with WebLinks: A Guidebook for Nutrition, 98/99,* are indexed at the back of the book. Sites are listed alphabetically by site name. The index can be used to find sites quickly, or for cross-reference.

# Morton Publishing Company

925 W. Kenyon Ave., Unit 12, Englewood, CO 80110
1-800-348-3777

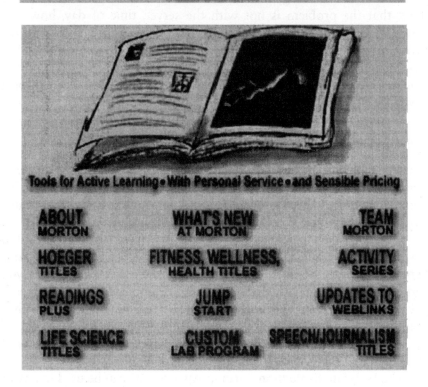

Tools for Active Learning • With Personal Service • and Sensible Pricing

**ABOUT** MORTON

**WHAT'S NEW** AT MORTON

**TEAM** MORTON

**HOEGER** TITLES

**FITNESS, WELLNESS, HEALTH TITLES**

**ACTIVITY** SERIES

**READINGS** PLUS

**JUMP** START

**UPDATES TO** WEBLINKS

**LIFE SCIENCE** TITLES

**CUSTOM** LAB PROGRAM

**SPEECH/JOURNALISM** TITLES

about morton publishing | fitness, wellness, health titles | life science titles
activity series | readingsplus | what's new at morton publishing | custom lab program
jumpstart | hoeger titles | updates to weblinks | team morton | speech/journalism titles

home | e-mail

# Be A Filter, Not a Sponge: Suggestions for Critical Thinking

Information. More is always better. Soak it up, like a sponge. The more you have, the smarter you are. Right?

Wrong!

Information does not necessarily equal knowledge. Information is only as good as how it is processed and evaluated—or filtered—by your brain, much like a coffee filter allows the rich liquid to seep through (the good stuff) and holds back the used coffee grounds (the dregs).

Filtering information is the basis of critical thinking. In other words, be a filter, not a sponge!

Critical thinking allows you to draw real knowledge out of information. But this does not happen by accident. To think critically, you must participate in what you see, read, and hear.

In other words, to think critically, you must think actively. You must question what you see and hear. You must listen to the responses to your questions and evaluate them with care. Then you must question again. And, perhaps, again. (A word of warning: with thousands of bits of information bombarding us daily, some things should just be ignored. Be discerning. Eliminate clutter.)

Questioning and listening are activities that come naturally to human beings. But doing them in ways that promote critical thinking is a skill that takes conscious effort and practice to develop and do well.

It is a worthwhile skill, though. And you can and should apply it to all aspects of your life, not just to what you read and study for your courses. It can help you to become better informed about the world, and it can even help you to have more rewarding relationships.

## Questions, Questions, Questions

Who? What? When? Where? How?

Not all of these questions will apply to every piece of information, but one or more of them surely will. As an example, here are a few questions that you might ask about an article in your local newspaper on the health benefits of regular exercise:

☐ **Who?** Consider the source. Who wrote it? Was a staff reporter assigned simply to relay information from a new medical study? Is the article an interview with a personal trainer who might be enthusiastic but not provide much hard data? Or is the article a review of the 1996 U.S. Surgeon General's Report on Physical Activity and Health—a report that is based on decades of research on physical activity and health? Do you find the source reliable, or do you think you might be getting sloppy reporting or even intentional misinformation to sway you to some viewpoint? Considering the source will cause you to view information with a healthy skepticism.

- [ ] **Where?** Assess the placement of the article in the newspaper to help you figure out its point. Does it appear in the hard-news section? Or is it a chatty piece in a "living" section, indicating that it might not have much hard data—or value. You should always take into account the total context in which information appears.

- [ ] **What?** What is the significance of the information contained in the article? Is it timely? Does it have any special relevance to you? Or is the newspaper simply trying to fill some space with a fluff piece on a slow news day?

- [ ] **How?** How does the information compare to what you may already know about the health benefits of exercise? Comparing and contrasting new information you encounter against what you may have already learned in class is a good technique for developing your critical thinking skills.

## Case Study in Critical Thinking: On the World Wide Web

One evening you come across a Web site on acupuncture. At the site is an article praising this ancient Chinese method of treating disease and relieving pain. It explains that some people even go to acupuncturists in an effort to stop smoking or lose weight.

"The answer to my prayers!" you say to yourself. Sign me up! Then you realize that you need to think critically about this information. How reliable is it? To find out, you begin to ask some questions.

In this case, you learn that the Web site is written and paid for by a group of health practitioners who specialize in alternative medicine — treatments like acupuncture and chiropractic and massage therapy. You call the group and learn that acupuncture treatments are not inexpensive. Although you realize that the group has a vested interest in encouraging Web users to give acupuncture a try, you learn through several trusted friends that the group is well respected in your community. A librarian recommends a book on alternative health, and through further research, you learn that, although some conventional medical doctors dismiss acupuncture, others are convinced that it provides distinct health benefits. You also learn that some insurance companies agree and provide coverage for these types of treatment.

Eventually, you conclude that acupuncture is something you want to learn more about and eventually try.

## Follow Up—and Be True to Yourself

As the case study shows, it is important to actively follow up. In checking the information on acupuncture, for example, you looked beyond the original Web site. You found other documents, you talked to friends, you contacted the holistic health group. You didn't rely on just one source to help you form an opinion. This sort of follow-up is essential to developing your critical thinking skills.

You also were true to yourself. Although you found no hard statistics proving beyond a shadow of a doubt that acupuncture works, you were open to considering that such alternative treatments have real health benefits. By contrast, someone who thinks that alternative medicine is hogwash will probably conclude from the exact same information that acupuncture does not work.

That's O.K. The point of critical thinking is not the conclusion, because rarely does any issue have clear "yes" and "no" answers. The valuable point is that you made the effort to think something through and develop an informed opinion. It is inevitable that your own values and goals will come into play, but critical thinking will help you learn to keep an open mind—to be open to new ideas and viewpoints.

## Be Involved

Critical thinking does not assess only what is said. It also considers what is *not* said. Look and listen for what is suggested or implied rather than overtly stated. In so doing, you interact with the material: You involve yourself in learning and thinking.

Through this process, you are empowered. Even though you may not be an expert on a subject, you can be an intelligent questioner and evaluator.

So, the next time that you come across an intriguing piece of information, remember: Who? What? When? Where? How? . . .

## Learn More About It: Resources

You may want to consider taking a course in critical thinking. Learning how to ask good questions and knowing how to evaluate information is an important skill, particularly as the amount of information available to the average person keeps expanding. Here are are a few print and online resources:

## IN PRINT

M. Neil Browne and Stuart M. Keeley, *Asking the Right Questions: A Guide to Critical Thinking*, 2nd ed. (Prentice-Hall, 1986).

Vicent Ryan Ruggiero, *Becoming a Critical Thinker*, 2nd ed. (Houghton Mifflin, 1996).

Glen Thomas and Gaye Smooth, "Critical Thinking: A Vital Work Skill," *Trust for Educational Leadership* (February/March 1994), pp. 34-38.

## ONLINE

### Effective Learning: Study Skills/Critical Thinking

http://www.cdtl.nus.sg/UFM/Effect/Es4_3_7.html

The National University of Singapore has a portion of its Web site devoted to student study skills, including critical thinking skills. This address will take you to several lively pages that define critical thinking, explain the characteristics of a critical thinker, and review fallacies to avoid. Although there are no links, the straightforward, practical text is well-designed and the guidelines are useful. (You might also want to check out the entire orientation section, which offers advice on how to make a smooth transition to higher education and on how to develop communication skills and time management skills, among other suggestions.)

### The Critical Thinking Community

http://www.sonoma.edu/CThink/

This site is maintained by Sonoma State University's Center for Critical Thinking. Site provides educators, students, and the public with a wealth of information about the theory and practice of critical thinking, concepts and definitions, techniques for learning and teaching, and classroom exercises that implement the principles. Other features include weekly updates, an Educator's Resource Guide for integrating critical thinking into the curriculum, a collection of critical thinking articles, and a list of conferences. Links to online discussion groups. The site is directed by Richard Paul, Ph.D., and comments are invited thru E-mail addresses provided. Also offers links to a sampling of critical thinking offices nationwide.

### Mission: Critical

http://www.sjsu.edu:80/depts/itl/

This site is produced by the Institute for Teaching and Learning at San Jose State University. Its goal is to create a "virtual lab" capable of familiarizing users with the basic concepts of critical thinking in a self-paced, interactive environment. Comments and reactions are encouraged, and an E-mail address is provided. Site includes links to each step in the process plus exercises for the student to do. A good online way to become a critical thinker.

# Using the World Wide Web as a Resource

These days it sometimes seems as if all we hear about is the World Wide Web. Web addresses are everywhere (in TV ads, magazines, newspapers, even some textbooks). Magazines on the Web are displayed in newsstand windows, and books about the Web appear in specially marked sections of every bookstore. Your college or university might even have its own Web site, or perhaps has plans to build one soon. What's the big appeal?

By sitting at a computer that has an Internet connection and a graphical browser for accessing the Web, we have at our fingertips a worldwide storehouse of information. We can search the Web to find information on just about anything. Need current information for a term paper on cancer prevention, women's health issues, nutritional supplements . . . ? Find it on the Web. Want to keep up with the gossip about the stars on your favorite soap, the latest statistics on an NFL team, your favorite group, news of the day? Find it on the Web. Interested in alternative health, school loans, the latest government report on physical activity and health? Find it on the Web. No matter the topic, it's in there. Why is the Web so useful?

The big draw of the Web is the way it links documents together. Imagine that you are reading a book and the author mentions another book. Because it sounds so interesting, you hop in your car and drive to the library. It's out for two more weeks. Frustrated, you head off to a bookstore. They don't have it in stock—but they could get it within a few days. Finally, you call a few other bookstores until you find one that has the book. You get back home, read a few pages, and this book refers to a favorite movie of yours. Because it's a favorite, you've got it on tape. You pop it into the VCR and watch it for a while. Then you decide to go back to reading the first book that started this burst of activity.

This is the sort of experience you can have when you're cruising the Web, and you never have to leave your chair! On the Web you can find documents that draw together text, graphics, and even sound and video. And when an author creates a document on the Web, it can contain links (highlighted text called hypertext) to any other Web document. When you click on these links, the new document is opened. A single Web page can contain links to pages from all over the world—and there are literally billions of pages on the Web. (However, not all pages contain links.)

So the World Wide Web is the part of the Internet with colorful graphics and hypertext—highlighted words that link you to related information elsewhere on the Web at the click of a mouse. In theory, it is a grand collection of documents from all around the world that you can navigate seamlessly. But how do you find what you're looking for among the billions of pages on the Web? And what should you look out for when you land at a Web site?

## Maneuvering Around the Web

If you have time to surf the Web and are not particular about where you end up, an online search engine or directory can be a useful tool. Online directories or search engines are Web sites that index and classify other Web sites. The drawback to using them is time, and there is no guarantee that the sites that have been indexed and classified are in good working order or contain credible, reliable information. Here is a list of the most popular search engines:

### Directories

**Alta Vista: Main Page**
http://www.altavista.digital.com

**Lycos Home Page**
http://www.lycos.com

**Excite**
http://www.excite.com

**Yahoo!**
http://www.yahoo.com

**Infoseek**
http://www.infoseek.com

### Using Web Addresses

Another method for working your way around the Web is to use a guidebook, such as this publication, *JumpStart with WebLinks: A Guidebook for Nutrition, 98/99*. In this guidebook, you have been provided with addresses of specific sites, which have been organized and categorized, and are appropriate for academic use. *JumpStart with WebLinks* gives you a specific address (http://. . .), which you can carefully type into the Location bar on your screen while you're online and using a graphical browser. (The most widely-used and best known browsers are Netscape and Mosaic, and both are available for free.) By going directly to a Web site using the site address, you know something about your starting point for navigating the Web. The starting point is a valid site, and you are able to make the most of your time on the Web. If you care to do more searching, you can take it from there.

## Some Helpful Hints

The Web is an increasingly relevant and effective source for up-to-date information. The best way to learn about it is to get online and experiment. Here are some helpful hints to avoid wasting time:

- Be precise; exactness of address counts.
- Get in the habit of notating sites that you want to refer to in the future. (For example, note the address, of course, and perhaps the date you visited the site. Note the subject matter at the site or briefly describe it. Note its audience, the geographic location, the organization that runs or sponsors the site, and any special features.)
- Use very specific key words when you are searching at a site or on the Web.
- Restrain yourself from carefully reading everything; know when to scroll and skim.
- Turn off the graphics if you want to speed up.
- Avoid "bookmarking" everything under the sun. (The Bookmark function allows you to save a site for future reference. However, for a variety of reasons, you're not always going to want to do that at the computer you are using to access the Web. A print record of particularly key sites can be easily shared with others, and is easily carried into class, etc. The "Making Your Own Connections" feature in this book can be used for saving and sharing key sites.)

## Glossary of Terms

Use the following definitions as an abbreviated introductory guide to terms to help you get a grip on what you are doing on the Web.

**back button:** allows you to retrace your hypersteps one link at a time.

**browsers:** tools for navigating around the Web.

**cyberspace:** loosely, a term that describes the world of information available through computer networks.

**directory:** a search engine—a "map" of items on the Web, such as is provided by Yahoo!, Excite, and Lycos.

**document:** anything from straight text on a topic (or business, or whatever) to information with multimedia elements.

**E-mail:** electronic mail; messages that flash instantaneously from one computer to another at the touch of a button (once you know how).

**hypertext:** a hyperlink that is a word; a highlighted visible word that you can click on to link to another document; selecting a link in one document immediately moves you into another.

**Internet:** a worldwide network of computer networks; it can be used to send and receive E-mail, read news, send and receive files, and connect to the Web.

**online:** loosely, being connected with other computer systems.

**online service:** America On-Line, CompuServe, etc.; companies that provide access to the Internet and additional services.

**multimedia:** a combination of different elements, such as text, pictures, and sound.

**search engines:** directories; online services (such as Yahoo!) that help you maneuver around the Web.

**Web (World Wide Web, or WWW):** a vast collection of documents that provides links from site to site and to related documents or sections or documents; a single Web page might contain links to pages from all over the world; it presents information in a familiar, booklike way. The Web is not the Internet; it is a part of the Internet—in fact, the most popular part—that makes the Net easier to use.

**Web site:** an individual location on the Web; any single site might consist of many pages.

## Resources for the Web

Here are two basic books:

Brad Hill, *World Wide Web Searching for Dummies* (IDG Books, 1997)

Jim Minatel, *Easy World Wide Web with Netscape* (Que, 1995)


Here are a few online resources:

**The Argus Clearinghouse: The Internet's Premier Research Library**
http://www.clearinghouse.net/

You will find definitions and explanations of the Internet at this site. Site also offers guides to Internet sites on a variety of topics, including nutrition and health.

**About the Internet**
http://home.netscape.com/assist/about_the_internet.html

A general introduction to the Internet and WWW and the features of Netscape—a superior, widely used graphical browser.

# Athletics/Fitness & Nutrition ▇ 1

What are the most important things an athlete needs to know about nutrition for optimal performance? According to Paul Saltman, a professor of biology at the University of California at San Diego, there are at least six important rules all athletes should know. (Source: "Six Nutrition Rules to Live By," *Women's Sports & Fitness*, November/December 1996.) The first of these is getting enough liquid to maintain hydration and the body's electrolyte balance. Although non-athletes can function on eight cups of fluid per day, athletes need more. Athletes working out in hot and humid weather may need to weigh themselves before and after an athletic event. For every pound lost, the athlete should consume two cups of fluid.

For most athletes, carbohydrates are the most important fuel. These are found in foods with starches; for example, bread, pasta and rice, fruits and fruit juices. (Source: "Alternative Energy Sources for Athletes," *Women's Sport and Fitness*, January/February 1997.)

Dietary fat is another important fuel. A majority of the calories athletes use during peak performance come from stored body fat. Eating excessive fat is unhealthy and unnecessary because protein, carbohydrates, and fat can all be stored as fat by the body. A few studies have found that highly trained endurance athletes may perform well on a high fat intake, but most sports nutritionists and trainers recommend high carbohydrate diets. (Source: "High Fat Diets Help Athletic Performance," *Science News*, May 4, 1996.)

To maximize the body's use of oxygen, B vitamins are needed. These include $B_6$, $B_{12}$, and folic acid. Minerals such as iron, copper, and other trace elements are important and can be found in red meat, fortified breakfast cereals, or supplements. Do athletes need supplements? Generally, a well-planned diet with adequate fluids can meet the needs of most athletes.

Intensive exercise causes muscle to break down. To restore muscle and help the body preserve its lean tissue, quality protein food is needed. In general, most athletes eating a typical American diet can get adequate protein. Excessive protein is not recommended because it can lead to excessive thirst and it's not an efficient fuel for the body. Uncooked protein foods such as raw eggs are never recommended because they can harbor harmful microbes. Good sources of protein include meat, fish and poultry, dried beans, eggs, and dairy products, which are excellent sources of calcium and vitamin D. Athletes need adequate calcium and vitamin D to help keep their bones strong.

# Athletics/Fitness & Nutrition

 Why do athletes need more fluid than nonathletes? • Why should athletes avoid raw meat or eggs? • Which nutrients are most important for athletes?

## ⚫WebLinks

**Gatorade Sports Science Institute**     **No. 1**

⚫ http://www.gssiweb.com/

The Gatorade Sports Science Institute provides information targeted towards athletic trainers, physicians, coaches, nutritionists, and anyone interested in sports medicine, sports nutrition, and exercise science. Visitors to the site can find out what's new in these fields, browse a list of interesting facts, post questions for response, and review the explanations to FAQs. Look for links to related topics.

**Nutrition and the Athlete from the University of Nebraska Extension**     **No. 2**

⚫ http://www.ianr.unl.edu/pubs/NebFacts/nf92-66.htm

This site focuses on the eating habits of athletes. Although there are no graphics or links, sensible nutrition guidelines for pre and post game are presented by Linda Boeckner, University of Nebraska Extension nutrition specialist.

**Penn State Sports Medicine Newsletter Homepage**     **No. 3**

⚫ http://cac.psu.edu/~hgk2/index.html

Articles from the *Penn State Sports Medicine Newsletter* are featured at this all-text site. The newsletter, a monthly publication of the Center for Sports Medicine at Pennsylvania State University, is written for a general audience and includes up-to-date, authoritative information on sports safety, sports nutrition, and exercise for general health. No links are available; however, information is provided on how to subscribe to, or receive previous issues of, the newsletter.

**The Physician and Sports Medicine Online**     **No. 4**

⚫ http://www.physsportsmed.com/index.html

Read about nutrition, exercise, injury prevention, and fitness at this site from Physician and Sports Medicine Online, a division of The McGraw-Hill Companies. Links provide access to the cover stories, abstracts from the current issue, and articles from previous issues. Visit their resource center or send questions for more information via e-mail.

**Shape Up America**     **No. 5**

⚫ http://www2.shapeup.org/sua/

Shape Up America, a brainchild of former surgeon general C. Everett Koop, offers credible, science-based health messages on nutrition, weight management, and physical fitness. Visit the BMI [Body Mass Index] Center, the Cyberkitchen, the Media Center, and the Professional Center Library. A list of general information is available for browsing.

# Athletics/Fitness & Nutrition

## Making Your Own Connections

**Address/URL**

Notes/Observations/
Site Description

http://
_____

_____

_____

_____


http://
_____

_____

_____

_____


http://
_____

_____

_____

_____


http://
_____

_____

_____

_____

# Athletics/Fitness & Nutrition

## Making Your Own Connections

Address/URL

http://
_____
_____
_____

http://
_____
_____
_____

http://
_____
_____
_____

http://
_____
_____
_____

# Cancer ▬▬▬▬▬▬▬▬▬▬▬ 2

One of the most significant ways to prevent many cancers is to adopt positive health habits, which include avoidance of tobacco, minimal exposure to ultraviolet rays, and a diet rich in fruits, vegetables, whole grains, and nonfat dairy products. Although these recommendations are endorsed by the American Cancer Society and many other groups, the role of diet in the development of cancer is not entirely understood. Some studies have linked diets high in fat and alcohol and low fiber to cancer. Smoked, preserved, or charred meats, and diets low in vitamins A and C, are thought by some scientists to also pose a risk for the disease. (Source: "New American Cancer Society Guidelines on Diet, Nutrition and Cancer Prevention," *Journal of the National Cancer Institute*, February 5, 1997.)

Eating more fruits, vegetables, and whole grains is generally sound advice, but many investigations into the diet and cancer connection are contradictory, or target only one food or a component of a food. For instance, a recent article claimed that drinking wine, which contains phenolic compounds, may delay the onset of cancer. (Source: "Study Finds Wine May Delay Onset of Cancer," *Cancer Weekly Plus*, December 9, 1996.) However, the *Journal of the National Cancer Institute* recently ran an article that links alcohol with the onset of cancer.

How does diet actually affect the development of cancer? Cancers develop after cancer-causing agents enter body cells and alter the cells' genetic material. In some instances, these altered cells begin to multiply uncontrollably, a process known as promotion. The most likely role for food as a cause of cancer is of promotion.

Some foods or food components that are suspected promoters include certain fats and oils, alcohol, and smoked foods. Foods or nutrients that appear to function as anti-promoters include calcium, fiber, the B vitamin folic acid, and vitamins and minerals known as antioxidants. Other components of food known as phytochemicals, indoles, protease inhibitors, and others all appear to function as anticancer agents. Where are these substances found? Fruits, vegetables, whole grains and nonfat dairy. Eating these foods as the foundation of the diet should ensure adequate intake of important anti-cancer compounds.

# Cancer

 Are anti-promoters found in vitamin supplements? • Why do so many articles appear to contradict each other? • Why are so many people ready to believe every news article they read?

## ●WebLinks

### American Cancer Society                                                No. 6
● http://www.cancer.org

Look for the latest cancer news, research progress, programs, events, available publications, and other resources. A special section provides details on tobacco and its association with the illness. Local and national societies can be accessed through the site.

### Cancer Prevention and Control Program                                 No. 7
● http://www.cdc.gov/nccdphp/dcpc/dcpchome.htm

The Cancer Prevention and Control Program is part of the Center for Chronic Disease Prevention and Health Promotion, a division of the Centers for Disease Control and Prevention. This homepage features current program fact sheets, publications, and related resources. Questions about the program may be submitted.

### Cancer Research Foundation of America                                  No. 8
● http://www.preventcancer.org/

The Cancer Research Foundation of America is committed to the prevention of cancer through education, smoking cessation, and dietary changes. Useful data is provided on reducing risk, preventable cancers, community outreach and prevention, science and research. A kid's corner is included.

### National 5 a Day                                                       No. 9
● http://www.dcpc.nci.nih.gov/5aday/

Five a Day for Better Health is a national nutrition program sponsored by the National Cancer Institute. It is designed to encourage Americans to eat five or more servings of fruits and vegetables every day. Links take you through the site, which presents details about the fruit and vegetable industries, recipes and tips, and corresponding state programs.

### Oncolink - Diet and Cancer                                            No. 10
● http://oncolink.upenn.edu/causeprevent/diet/index.html

Maintained by the University of Pennsylvania Cancer Center, this broad site is a good place to start when researching the relationship of diet to cancer. It contains information on fluoridated water and artificial sweeteners. Links to related sites —including the National Cancer Institute, Cable News Network, Reuters, Scientific American, USA Today—and a list of fast food fat contents serve as valuable resources.

# Making Your Own Connections

| Address/URL | Notes/Observations/Site Description |
|---|---|

http://
_____
_____
_____

http://
_____
_____
_____

http://
_____
_____
_____

http://
_____
_____
_____

## Making Your Own Connections

| Address/URL | Notes/Observations/Site Description |
|---|---|
| http:// | |
| http:// | |
| http:// | |
| http:// | |

# Cardiovascular Disease 3

Heart disease is the leading cause of death for both men and women in the United States. As a result, there have been numerous studies to attempt to determine its causes. It is known that smoking, lack of exercise, obesity, elevated serum cholesterol, and diet all play a role in the development of heart disease, although the role of diet and serum cholesterol are somewhat unclear. For years, nutritionists have urged people to eat a lowfat diet to help lower serum cholesterol and reduce the risk of heart disease. A government funded study called the Multiple Risk Factor Intervention Trial (MRFIT) found that lowering blood cholesterol resulted in a trivial decrease in deaths from heart disease. A second study, the Lipid Research Clinics Coronary Primary Prevention Trial, also failed to relate lowered serum cholesterol and a reduced death rate. (Source: "Diet and Heart Disease: Not What You Think," *Consumers' Research Magazine*, June 1996.)

Dietary components linked to heart disease include a high intake of fat and low consumption of fruits and vegetables. However, the exact nature of the relationship of fat and heart disease is unclear. During the past 70 years, the use of vegetable fats in this country has increased, especially hydrogenated or hardened fats in the form of margarine and shortening. Forty years ago researchers found that eating these foods, which contain trans fatty acids, increased the risk of heart disease. (Source: "Why Butter Is Good For You," *Consumers' Research Magazine*, March 1996.) Scientists also have found that an excess of vegetables oils, even if they are not hardened, seem to play a role in causing heart disease because they affect hormones that play a role in various chemical processes in the body.

The role of fruits and vegetables is less confusing. Researchers have determined that a deficiency of vitamins $B_6$, $B_{12}$, and folate lead to hardening of the arteries and the buildup of plaque. While $B_{12}$ is found almost exclusively in animal products, $B_6$ and folate are found in fruits and vegetables. (Source: "Are You Getting Enough Folate?," *Healthline*, February 1996.) Fruits and vegetables are also a source of dietary fiber and vitamin C. Vitamin C makes arterial walls less likely to become inflamed, and helps maintain the integrity of both heart muscle and blood vessels. Dietary fiber appears to help lower serum cholesterol. (Source: "High Fiber Diet and Heart Disease," *Harvard Heart Letter*, June 1996.)

Overall, a diet rich in fruits and vegetables, whole grains, and lowfat animal proteins may help protect against heart disease. Regular exercise and no smoking are also important. Merely reducing fats or switching from butter to margarine in an attempt to lower serum cholesterol may not be beneficial and may even be harmful.

# Cardiovascular Disease

**?** What vitamins are thought to play a role in the prevention of heart disease? • What substances in shortening and margarine may be harmful? • What is the role of vitamin C in the prevention of heart disease?

## ⬤WebLinks

### American Heart Association Food and Nutrition                    No. 11
⬤ http://207.211.141.25/

Search the American Heart Association's homepage for reliable information and the latest news. Browse their heart and stroke A–Z guide, access your local chapter, and send questions or messages. Look for the association's diet eating plan and the recipe of the month. Includes an Interactive Risk Assessment.

### Cardiovascular Information                    No. 12
⬤ http://www.nhlbi.nih.gov/nhlbi/cardio/cardio.htm

This easy-to-navigate site is maintained by the National Heart, Lung, and Blood Institute. It presents no-nonsense information on a variety of topics, including high blood pressure, cholesterol, obesity, heart attack, and other cardiovascular issues. Links are provided to related documents.

### Healthy Eating for Health Living                    No. 13
⬤ http://www.fi.edu/biosci/healthy/diet.html

Search this site for guidelines on what and how much to eat based on the food pyramid and the basic food groups. Look for heart smart hints, diet resources, and links to other topics such as healthy eating tips for children and adults and information on antioxidants and cholesterol.

### Step by Step: Eating to Lower Your High Blood Cholesterol                    No. 14
⬤ http://www.nih.gov/news/

The National Institutes of Health presents the latest news and information. Look for press releases and upcoming events. Lots of links lead to more detailed pages.

## Making Your Own Connections

Address/URL

Notes/Observations/
Site Description

http://
_____
_____
_____
_____

http://
_____
_____
_____
_____

http://
_____
_____
_____
_____

http://
_____
_____
_____
_____

# Cardiovascular Disease

## Making Your Own Connections

Address/URL

Notes/Observations/
Site Description

http://

_____

_____

_____

http://

_____

_____

_____

http://

_____

_____

_____

http://

_____

_____

_____

# Chronic Diseases 4

Each year, over a million people in this country suffer a bone fracture attributable to osteoporosis, making the disease one of the most common of the chronic, degenerative diseases. Osteoporosis is one of many illnesses related to diet and nutrition status, which also include liver diseases, digestive conditions, kidney diseases, and others. Inadequate nutrition is not the specific cause of these conditions, but it contributes to or exacerbates them. In some cases, a proper diet is necessary to manage these diseases, or diet may help to relieve symptoms.

Osteoporosis, which affects the majority of women over age 75, has few or no symptoms at its onset. The disease causes the loss of minerals in bone, which increases the risk of fracture. Risk factors include heredity, lack of exercise, being underweight, smoking, alcohol use, excessive protein and sodium intake, and lack of calcium, vitamin D, and fluoride. Recently, researchers from the University of Illinois have found that diets rich in soy foods, such as tofu, soy milk, and soy flour, may help fight osteoporosis. Although the investigators hoped to find that soy would help prevent bone loss in older women, they actually saw a small increase in density and bone mineral content of the small of the back, a spot prone to bone loss and fractures. Soy foods contain isoflavones, which are weak, plant version of estrogen and may help prevent bone loss. (Source: "Want Better Bones? Ah Soy," *Prevention*, January 1997.)

Eating soy and calcium may help prevent osteoporosis, but the relationship between diet and arthritis is less clear. Millions of arthritis sufferers turn to unproven treatments, dietary or otherwise, to ease the pain of their inflamed joints. A recent study has shown that vitamins may offer some relief, though no food has been shown to cure arthritis. Vitamin D and fish oils, which contain vitamins D and E, have been shown to offer some benefits. (Source: "Fish Oils Shine in New Arthritis Study," *Environmental Nutrition*, October 1996.)

Eating fish oils and soy may impact arthritis and osteoporosis. For liver and kidney diseases, diet can help manage these conditions. Kidney patients, for instance, are often on diets that restrict their intake of protein, potassium, and other nutrients. For patients suffering various digestive ailments, diet can make a difference. Millions of people in this country take antacids to relieve heartburn and gastrointestinal distress. These drugs can reduce iron absorption and increase calcium and phosphorus excretion. For many people, eating smaller, more frequent meals that are lower in fat may prevent these digestive upsets.

# Chronic Diseases

 What foods are recommended to help prevent osteoporosis? • Why are soy foods thought to be beneficial? • How can dietary changes affect heartburn?

# ⊘Web*Links*

### Alphabetical Disease Site                                      No. 15
⊘ http://www.mic.ki.se/Diseases/alphalist.html

Presented by the Karolinska Institute Library and Information Center, this page lists hundreds of diseases and disorders. Scan the list for a particular entry or click on a letter to review a certain section. This is a simple way to access details on specific illnesses and ailments.

### Crohns Disease/Ulcerative Colitis Home Page                   No. 16
⊘ http://qurlyjoe.bu.edu/cduchome.html

This site presents excerpts from relevant publications, new research results, and information from medical institutions, pharmaceutical companies, and service providers. E-mail addresses to obtain answers to FAQs are also provided. Useful links available.

### National Institute of Diabetes and Digestive
### and Kidney Diseases (NIDDK)                                    No. 17
⊘ http://www.niddk.nih.gov/NIDDK_HomePage.html

News and information for researchers, professionals, and the general public on diabetes, digestive diseases, endocrine and metabolic diseases, kidney diseases, nutrition, obesity, and urologic diseases are provided at this site by the NIDDK, a division of the National Institutes of Health. Many links pertaining to the topics are available.

### National Osteoporosis Foundation                              No. 18
⊘ http://www.nof.org/

This organization is America's leading resource for up-to-date, medically sound information on the cause, prevention, detection, and treatment of osteoporosis. Tabs throughout the site lead to data on risk factors and bone health. A flashing tab directs a visitor to cutting edge reports and extensive statistics. A multitude of links provides further details and access to a related site.

## Making Your Own Connections

**Address/URL**

Notes/Observations/
Site Description

http:// _____

_____

_____

_____

http:// _____

_____

_____

_____

http:// _____

_____

_____

_____

http:// _____

_____

_____

_____

## *Making Your Own Connections*

**Address/URL**

**Notes/Observations/
Site Description**

http://

_____

_____

_____

http://

_____

_____

_____

http://

_____

_____

_____

http://

_____

_____

_____

# Community Nutrition Programs ▪ 5

Several government-based programs take aim at preventing or relieving domestic hunger, providing meals, and disseminating nutrition information. These programs include Food Stamps, the Special Supplemental Program for Women, Infants, and Children (WIC), and Title IIIC for seniors.

The Food Stamp program, administered by the U. S. Department of Agriculture (USDA), issues food stamp coupons through state social service agencies to low-income individuals and households. Recipients may use the coupons as cash to buy edible groceries, but not non-food items such as tobacco, paper products, and cleaning items. More than 27 million people in this country receive food stamps at a cost of over $22 billion per year. (Source: "Hungrier in America," *America*, May 18, 1996.) Although food stamps are an income supplement, there is no nutrition education component.

The WIC program, also sponsored by the USDA, provides nutrition support to low-income women at nutritional risk who are pregnant or who have infants or preschool children. (Source: "WIC Nutrition Risk Criteria," *Nutrition Today*, October 1996.) WIC offers vouchers redeemable for specific foods, which supply the nutrients most important for growth and development. WIC, unlike food stamps, offers nutrition education to recipients. It has been proven effective in reducing health care costs and incidences of low birth weight, as well as other medical problems. (Source: "Twenty Years of WIC: A Review of Some Effects of the Program," *Journal of the American Dietetics Association*, July 1997.)

Other programs that provide food include the school breakfast and lunch programs, the Summer Food Service, the Child and Adult Care programs, and nutrition programs for older Americans. The Title IIIC program offers seniors a nutritious lunch as well as activities and socialization. There are also government programs for American Indian reservations and Puerto Rico.

Despite the government's efforts, federal programs that provide food to the needy are not completely successful due to budget cuts and the increased demand for food aid. In an effort to help the hungry where government programs fall short, local communities have responded with private efforts. Through community-based agencies and religious organizations, soup kitchens and shelters provide food to the hungry. Food pantries and community vegetable gardens also contribute groceries to those in need. These efforts provide emergency relief, though they do not address the greater long-term problem of maintaining food security for all Americans.

# Community Nutrition Programs

What items are redeemable for food stamps? • What government programs benefit school children? • Which programs offer nutrition education in addition to food benefits. • What are some of the major benefits of the WIC program? • Why are government programs falling short of providing food for all needy Americans? • What can local communities do to impact the situation when government efforts falter?

## ●WebLinks

**Brown University's Hunger Web**　　　　　　　　　　　　　**No. 19**

● http://www.brown.edu/Departments/World_Hunger_Program/

The first of its kind in this format, this site is dedicated to providing information about world hunger. Research, field work, and details on advocacy, policy, education, and training are presented by Brown University.

**Food Stamp Program**　　　　　　　　　　　　　　　　**No. 20**

● http://www.usda.gov/fcs/fs.htm

What's new in food stamps and welfare reform, details on food stamp rights and information about Electronic Benefits Transfer (EBT) are addressed at this brief site. Links to the Food and Nutrition Information Center are available.

**Healthy School Meals Resource System**　　　　　　　　　**No. 21**

● http://schoolmeals.nal.usda.gov:8001/team.html

From the U.S. Department of Agriculture (USDA), this site offers a database of training materials, a multimedia corner, and an interactive forum called "Meal Talk" specifically for professionals operating Child Nutrition Programs, the USDA's school meals initiative for healthy children. Information on community nutrition action programs and a collection of food services resources on the Web can also be found. Valuable links connect a visitor to other sites, including the Food and Nutrition Information Center, Dietary Guidelines for Americans, and the USDA food guide pyramid.

**Self Help and Resource Exchange (SHARE)**　　　　　　　**No. 22**

● http://www.meer.net/users/taylor/share.htm

This modest site lists addresses and phone numbers of organizations that deal with the northern California office of SHARE, a nationwide, nonprofit association that enables people to obtain food in an atmosphere of human dignity.

**WIC Program**　　　　　　　　　　　　　　　　　　　**No. 23**

● http://www.usda.gov/

The U.S. Department of Agriculture provides information about the agency and its programs. Link to the latest news and information from this homepage.

# Community Nutrition Programs

## Making Your Own Connections

**Address/URL**

**Notes/Observations/
Site Description**

http://
_____
_____
_____
_____

http://
_____
_____
_____
_____

http://
_____
_____
_____
_____

http://
_____
_____
_____
_____

# Community Nutrition Programs

## Making Your Own Connections

| Address/URL | Notes/Observations/Site Description |
|---|---|
| http:// | |
| http:// | |
| http:// | |
| http:// | |

# Dental Health Nutrition

Dental decay is a serious health concern that afflicts nearly everyone in this country, half by the time they are two years old. Although fluoridation of drinking water has reduced the incidence of cavities, sugar, baby formula, and heredity all play a role. Cavities develop as acids produced by bacteria grow in the mouth and erode tooth enamel. Bacteria build colonies, or plaque, whenever they are able to establish themselves on the surface of the tooth. Once they become established, they increase and attach themselves more firmly to the tooth. Unless brushed, scraped or flossed away, the acids cause pits that turn into cavities. Plaque works below the gum line, too. Its acid damages the roots of teeth and the jawbone in which they are embedded, loosening teeth and leading to gum infections. Gum disease, which can cause tooth loss, is a problem for the majority of Americans by their later years. Fortunately, flossing every day reduces this risk.

Does sugar cause decay? The bacteria that cause cavities thrive on carbohydrates, including sugar and starch. The length of time sugar and starch come in contact with teeth, how sticky the food is, and how often it's eaten are especially important. Bacteria produce acid for up to 30 minutes after exposure to sugar. (Source: "Nutritional Role of Sugars in Oral Health," *American Journal of Clinical Nutrition*, Volume 62, 1995.) Some forms of candy, such as caramels, may be less harmful than previously believed because the sugar dissolves completely and is washed away in saliva. Particles from grain products, including cookies, cereals, and crackers, may be worse than once thought because they may get stuck in the teeth and do not dissolve. Brushing or rinsing the mouth after eating these foods can help prevent these particles from remaining in the mouth.

Sugary and starchy foods can cause cavities, but not everyone is aware of the decay-producing effects of milk. Babies, in particular, are at risk of dental decay related to milk consumption. Both milk and baby formula contain lactose, a naturally occurring sugar. Prolonged sucking on a bottle of milk or infant formula bathes the upper teeth in a sugar-rich liquid that enhances the growth of decay-causing bacteria. Some babies who are regularly put to bed with a bottle sometimes have their upper teeth decayed all the way to the gum line, a condition known as nursing bottle syndrome or baby bottle tooth decay. (Source: "Preventing the Baby Bottle Tooth Decay," *Public Health Reports,* January 1996.)

Other risks to dental enamel include sucking or chewing on chewable vitamin C tablets. These pills contain acids that can erode tooth enamel. (Source: "Chewable Vitamin C Bad for Teeth," *Environmental Nutrition*, March 1996.)

# Dental Health & Nutrition

 What foods can increase the risk of dental decay? • Why are carbohydrates a risk? • Why should babies not be put to bed with a bottle?

# ⊘WebLinks

### American Dental Association's (ADA) Diet and Dental Health        No. 24
⊕ http://www.ada.org/topics/diet.html

Consumer information, ADA news releases, and journal previews are among the topics covered at this site. Links provided take visitors to related pages.

### Dental Assist        No. 25
⊕ http://www.dentistry.com/assist.html

An interactive Q&A service about teeth is presented by Dr. Bill and Dr. Jeff. Links to tooth-related sites are included, as well as answers to specific questions. As sponsors of Aesthetic Dentistry Associates, Drs. Bill Langstaff, DDS, and Jeff Wissot, DDS, offer the opportunity to inquire about new advances in dental treatment options and to address related topics that may impact your dental care choices.

### National Institute of Dental Research: A Healthy Mouth for Your Baby   No. 26
⊕ http://www.nidr.nih.gov/pubs/hmouth/text.htm

Few links are provided but important information is furnished. Topics include checking and cleaning baby's teeth, feeding baby healthy food, preventing baby bottle tooth decay, protecting baby's teeth with fluoride, and taking a child to the dentist.

### Snack Smart for Healthy Teeth        No. 27
⊕ http://www.nidr.nih.gov/pubs/snaksmrt/main.htm

Obtain an explanation of why sugar snacks can be bad and how sugars attack your teeth from this site and its links. Don't miss the list of smart snack foods.

## Making Your Own Connections

| Address/URL | Notes/Observations/ Site Description |
|---|---|

http://
_____
_____
_____

http://
_____
_____
_____

http://
_____
_____
_____

http://
_____
_____
_____

# Dental Health & Nutrition

## Making Your Own Connections

| Address/URL | Notes/Observations/ Site Description |
|---|---|

http://
_____

_____

_____

_____


http://
_____

_____

_____

_____


http://
_____

_____

_____

_____


http://
_____

_____

_____

_____

# Diabetes     7

Diabetes can lead to or contribute to any number of other diseases. It is among the top 10 killers of adults and the leading cause of blindness in the Unites States. It kills more people each year than either breast cancer or AIDS and affects 16 million people. Although we should certainly be concerned with these numbers, the good news about diabetes is that at least 75 percent of the new cases of adult-onset diabetes can probably be prevented. (Source: "How to Avoid Adult Onset Diabetes," *Nutrition Action Health Letter,* September 1996.) Weight loss and exercise are the main defenses, and nutritional supplements, like chromium or vitamins C and E, may also make a difference. (Source: "Chromium's Promise Primarily for Diabetes," *Environmental Nutrition,* January 1997.)

Of the 16 million people with diabetes, close to 95 percent have Type II or adult-onset. The other form, juvenile onset, is really a different disease with a different cause and treatment. What causes adult diabetes and how can it be prevented? In addition to heredity, there are two primary dietary risk factors: obesity and lack of exercise. In a dozen studies that followed tens of thousands of people for years, being overweight increased the risk of developing the disease by more than tenfold. Although it's not exactly clear why being overweight increases the risk of diabetes, it is certain that losing some extra weight helps prevent the condition. And it's not just the extra weight that matters. Where the pounds are stored is also a risk factor. Being heavy in the middle appears to be a greater risk than weight below the waist. It seems that fat deposited in the upper body results in an abnormal use of insulin.

Dietary factors that can positively affect diabetes include chromium and antioxidants. Chromium seems to help reduce glucose levels in those who are not getting enough. This may postpone the onset of diabetes. Chromium supplements, however, only showed a modest benefit in a recent study, and it's not clear if its benefits last over time. Antioxidants appear to be more promising. Vitamin C, when given to diabetics, helped clear glucose from their blood. Studies on vitamin E have been mixed: Large doses for three months led to a drop in blood glucose levels for diabetics.

Does eating sugar cause diabetes? Sugar does not appear to cause the disease, and certain foods may help prevent it. High fiber foods including fruits, vegetables, beans (legumes), and whole grains are associated with a lower risk of diabetes. (Source: "Nutrition Notes," *Diabetes Forecast,* March 1997.)

# Diabetes

**?** What type of diabetes is most common? • How can diabetes be prevented? • What foods are linked to a reduced risk of diabetes? • What are the primary risk factors? • What role do vitamins play, if any? • What is the role of sugar in the development of diabetes?

## ●WebLinks

**Academy for the Advancement of Diabetes Research and Treatment**     No. 28

● http://drinet.med.miami.edu/

Many links provide access to topics and pages pertaining to diabetes research and treatment. Solid information is presented.

**American Diabetes Association**     No. 29

● http://www.diabetes.org/custom.asp

Interactive launch allows visitors the opportunity to customize their searches. Site offers diabetes information, research updates, Internet resources, risk factors, recipes, and volunteer and support opportunities. Additional links provided.

**Children and Diabetes**     No. 30

● http://www.castleweb.com/diabetes/

Loads of links and a search engine provide lots of easy-to-locate information. Learn about the basics of diabetes, food and diet issues, and available resources. Serves as an online community for individuals and families living with Type 1 diabetes.

**Reducing the Burden of Diabetes: Diabetes Articles from
the Centers for Disease Control and Prevention**     No. 31

● http://www.cdc.gov/nccdphp/ddt/abstract.htm

Links provide access to research articles and abstracts on diabetes. This site is maintained by the Centers for Disease Control and Prevention.

# Making Your Own Connections

| Address/URL | Notes/Observations/ Site Description |
|---|---|
| http://_____ _____ _____ _____ | |
| http://_____ _____ _____ _____ | |
| http://_____ _____ _____ _____ | |
| http://_____ _____ _____ _____ | |

## Making Your Own Connections

| Address/URL | Notes/Observations/ Site Description |
|---|---|
| http:// | |
| http:// | |
| http:// | |
| http:// | |

# Dieting & Weight Control

During the past 25 years, the number of men, women, and children in the United States who are overweight has been steadily increasing despite the number of people dieting and eating lowfat foods. Many people have been decreasing the fat content of their diets by eating nonfat ice cream, reduced fat cookies, and lowfat salad dressings. Unfortunately, we have also increased our intake of total calories and not adjusted our exercise patterns. It seems that the calories from all those reduced fat cookies are adding up! People eating fat-free foods may be eating more because they perceive these foods to be lower in calories, which is not always the case. (Source: "Is Your Diet Making You Fat," *Woman's Day,* April 22, 1997.) What should we eat? Experts recommend lowfat, low *calorie* foods like fruits, vegetables, and grains. These foods, unlike reduced fat cookies, also offer vitamins, minerals and fiber, which give us a feeling of being full.

Besides our diets, other reasons are contributing to the national weight gain. These include eating more meals away from home, lack of nutrition knowledge, and lack of exercise. Although all of these factors are controllable, we may also be gaining weight because of our genes. For some overweight individuals, inherited levels of hormones such as leptin may be a problem. Recent studies have shown that people with low levels of leptin are prone to weight gain. (Source: "Low Leptin Concentrations Linked to Weight Gain," *Lancet,* February 1, 1997.) Though we can't control our genes, most of us, fortunately, can lose weight through a combination of diet and exercise.

While Americans are getting fatter, the amount spent on weight loss products continues to climb. Currently, we spend $30 to 50 billion dollars each year on these mostly ineffective and potentially harmful products and services. The latest product, a fat substitute called olestra, was approved by the Food and Drug Administration for use in salted snacks and crackers. Olestra must carry a warning advising consumers that it may inhibit absorption of some vitamins and minerals and may cause cramps and loose stools, but Procter & Gamble, the maker of olestra, has gambled over $200 million that people will be willing to use it. (Source: John Nolan, "More Cramps, Less Filling: Olestra Label Will Be a Marketing Challenge," *USA Today,* January 31, 1996, p. C1.)

Millions of people use reduced calorie and fat products in largely unsuccessful attempts to lose weight. However, most experts believe that it is far better to prevent weight gain than to try to lose it after it has accumulated.

# Dieting & Weight Control

 Why are Americans getting heavier? • How does heredity affect weight? • Why are low fat foods not helping people to lose weight?

## ⬤WebLinks

**Dietary Guidelines for Americans**　　　No. 32

🌐 http://www.nalusda.gov/fnic/dga/dguide95.html

Every few years the U.S. Department of Agriculture modifies the national nutrition guidelines in response to new research. This site explains the current guidelines.

**Duke University: Diet & Fitness Center**　　　No. 33

🌐 http://dmi-www.mc.duke.edu/dfc/home.html

Weight management, lifestyle changes, and medical regulations are the focuses of this center at Duke University. The site presents answers to FAQs, success stories, recipes, and details on obesity genes. Links lead to other valuable material.

**Fast Food Facts—Interactive Food Finder**　　　No. 34

🌐 http://www.olen.com/food/

This interactive site from Olen Publishing Company provides various options for identifying nutrient information of foods at many of the popular fast food restaurants. It can also create a menu based on a specific nutritional profile. This information can help people make healthful choices at fast food restaurants.

**Patient Information Documents on Nutrition and Obesity**　　　No. 35

🌐 http://www.niddk.nih.gov/NutritionDocs.html

This is a government-sponsored site that has a list of diet and activity related topics—everything from binge eating to weight cycling. Therefore, it is a good site for exploring a wide range of weight management issues. You can also find national statistics about the prevalence of obesity here.

**Tips for Eating Out**　　　No. 36

🌐 http://www.ars.usda.gov/is/pr/eatout1196.htm

This site offers several interesting statistics about current eating trends based on a study conducted by The Food Surveys Research Group for the Agricultural Research Service. The results of the study are offered here as well as tips provided by the USDA for making healthier food choices.

**Weight Control Information Network (WIN)**　　　No. 37

🌐 http://www.niddk.nih.gov.NutritionDocs.html

Patient information on nutrition and obesity is presented by the National Institute of Diabetes and Digestive and Kidney Diseases, a division of the National Institutes of Health. An array of links connects to related information on binge eating disorder, dieting and gallstones, gastric surgery for severe obesity, physical activity and weight control, prescription medications for the treatment of obesity, and other topics.

# Dieting & Weight Control

## Making Your Own Connections

**Address/URL**

**Notes/Observations/
Site Description**

http://
_____
_____
_____

http://
_____
_____
_____

http://
_____
_____
_____

http://
_____
_____
_____

# Dieting & Weight Control

## Making Your Own Connections

| Address/URL | Notes/Observations/ Site Description |
|---|---|
| http:// | |
| http:// | |
| http:// | |
| http:// | |

# Drug Use ━━━━━━━━━━━━━ 9

Many legal and illegal drugs are used in this country, creating health, legal, and societal concerns. Many of these drugs also affect nutritional status in a variety of ways. For instance, stimulant drugs, whether legal or otherwise, speed up metabolism, cause insomnia, and suppress hunger. Stimulants such as caffeine can also act as a diuretic, causing the kidneys to work harder. The body also excretes large amounts of calcium when an excessive amount of caffeine is consumed. Caffeine, especially in large amounts, may also cause heart problems. (Source: "New Heart Risk From Too Much Coffee?" *Science News*, January 11, 1997.) Caffeine is found in coffee, non-herbal tea, cola, and some medications.

Nicotine, the addictive element is tobacco, is also a stimulant. Smoking affects nutritional status in many ways. For instance, studies have found that smokers eat differently than nonsmokers. (Source: "Food and Nutrient Intake Differences between Smokers and Non-smokers in the U.S.," *American Journal of Public Health*, Volume 80, 1990.) Smokers eat less fiber and foods rich in vitamins and minerals. This may be related to social and economic status, education, or different taste perceptions among smokers. Smokers also break down vitamin C faster than nonsmokers, so they need more of this vitamin. It is estimated that the vitamin C requirement of smokers may be twice as high as that of nonsmokers. A further nutritional difference between smokers and nonsmokers is related to body weight. In general, smokers have lower body weights than nonsmokers. When people quit smoking, they typically gain weight in response to several factors, including lowered metabolic rate, improved food tastes and eating rather than smoking. (Source: "Smoking Cessation Can Lead to Weight Gain," *Idea Today*, April 1996.) Exercising regularly after quitting smoking can help prevent weight gain.

Depressant drugs such as alcohol also affect nutritional status. The more alcohol a person drinks, the less likely he or she will eat a sufficient quantity of food to get adequate nutrition. Alcohol supplies the body with calories, but, like refined sugar, alcohol calories supply little or no nutrients. Alcohol also affects the body's ability to absorb vitamins and minerals, often leading to deficiencies. On the other hand, moderate amounts of alcohol, two or less drinks a day for men and one or less for women, can actually enhance health. Studies have shown that moderate drinking is beneficial to the heart and promotes "good" cholesterol.

# Drug Use

 What are the nutritional consequences of caffeine-containing beverages? • How does smoking affect weight and nutritional status? • What are the nutritional risks of excessive drinking?

## ⊘WebLinks

### Caffeine                                                    No. 38
⊘ http://h-devil-www.mc.duke.edu/h-devil/nutrit/caffeine.htm

This all-text page maintained by Duke University describes caffeine, a stimulant that causes increased heart rate and blood pressure. Tips on how to reduce caffeine in your diet, suggestions on who should avoid or limit caffeine, and major sources of caffeine are listed. Questions can be submitted for further exploration.

### Factline on Cocaine                                        No. 39
⊘ http://www.drugs.indiana.edu/pubs/factline/coke.html

Text, graphics, and links provide practical facts about cocaine. Look for data on cocaine hydrochloride, freebase cocaine, crack, and legal issues. The site is maintained by Indiana University's Prevention Resource Center.

### Health Hotlist                                             No. 40
⊘ http://sln.fi.edu/tfi/hotlists/health.html

Maneuver easily through the site to find details on caffeine, nutrition, drugs, alcohol, illnesses, and health facts. Each item has worthwhile links to related pages. Resources presented by the University of Michigan and the University of Arizona Health Sciences Library.

### Information on Drugs of Abuse                              No. 41
⊘ http://www.nida.nih.gov/DrugAbuse.html

The National Institute on Drug Abuse furnishes summaries of drug related issues, detailed data on many drugs, reliable statistics, and an alphabetical list of commonly abused drugs. Related links provide additional information.

### Tobacco Information & Prevention Sourcepage                No. 42
⊘ http://www.cdc.gov/tobacco/

This site is brought to you from the Centers of Disease Control and Prevention. Look for overview, in the news, research, educational materials, publications, resources, and FAQs. Also supplied are surgeon general's reports, tips on how to quit smoking, and messages to kids and teens.

### Web of Addictions: Tobacco                                No. 43
⊘ http;//www.well.com/user/woa/facts.htm#tobacco

This page is a branch of the Web of Addiction site. A list of links under the heading of tobacco is provided and includes Tobacco-IPRC (Indiana Prevention Resource Center at Indiana University), Smokeless Tobacco-MoDADA, Quitting Smokeless Tobacco-Alice, Cigarette Smoking-MODADA, Cigarette Smoking and Adults-Oncolink, and Health Facts about Tobacco-WHO. Great site with multiple links to other drugs as well as tobacco.

## Making Your Own Connections

Address/URL

Notes/Observations/
Site Description

http://
_____
_____
_____
_____

http://
_____
_____
_____
_____

http://
_____
_____
_____
_____

http://
_____
_____
_____
_____

## Making Your Own Connections

Address/URL

Notes/Observations/
Site Description

http://
_____
_____
_____

http://
_____
_____
_____

http://
_____
_____
_____

http://
_____
_____
_____

# Eating Disorders 10

According to recent data from the Centers for Disease Control and Prevention (CDC) in Atlanta, 63 percent of teenage girls are regular dieters. (Source: "Eating Disorders Awareness and Prevention," *Health Letter on the CDC*, February 17, 1997.) Although dieting doesn't always lead to an eating disorder, it is often a trigger. Currently, there are an estimated eight million Americans, mostly girls and women, suffering from various eating disorders. The vast majority suffer from compulsive overeating, which may be the most common form of eating disorder. (Source: "Dysfunctional Eating," *Healthy Weight Journal,* September/October 1996.) Compulsive overeaters, or binge eaters, may suffer from a condition similar to drug or alcohol addiction. What can begin as something pleasurable can turn into a serious problem, as eating becomes a food addiction. Those with a food addiction lose control over their eating much as an alcoholic may lose control over his or her drinking.

Some compulsive or binge eaters may develop bulimia, which is characterized by binge eating followed by either self-induced vomiting or laxative abuse. Bulimics, unlike anorexics who often look starved, do not look emaciated. Their weight may appear normal or even above normal. Bulimia is characterized by shame, guilt, or disgust with one's self after eating huge quantities of food. Anorexics are at risk for hormone imbalances, bone loss, and heart problems, while bulimics are at health risks related to frequent vomiting and purging. They may develop mineral imbalances, throat infections, and tooth decay from stomach acids coming into contact with their teeth. (Source: "Binge Eating Comes Out of the Closet," *Tufts Nutrition & Diet Newsletter,* January 1997.)

With so many physical and mental health problems associated with eating disorders, why do so many girls, women, and increasingly, men, develop these conditions? Risk factors include low self-esteem, negative body image, and family dysfunction. Eating disorders are complex and serious conditions that require professional treatment to avoid permanent physical and emotional damage. Treatment usually deals with the behavioral, physical, and psychological aspects of the disorder. Persons with eating disorders learn how to develop new and different eating patterns, and to understand and cope with the reasons behind the condition. The physical problems also need to be addressed with nutritional supplements and medication.

# Eating Disorders

 What are the health risks associated with bulimia? With anorexia? • What are the risk factors related to eating disorders?

## ●WebLinks

**American Academy of Child and Adolescent Psychiatry**     No. 44

● http://www.aacap.org/web/aacap/

The American Academy of Child and Adolescent Psychiatry presents research on children's mental health. "Facts for Families," which provides details on eating disorders and family concerns, is furnished. Links include a site search and breaking news. The site was honored as a 1995 Best Web Site, Top 5% Web Site, Grohol Best Web Site for Mental Health, and Web Site of the Month by Psychiatry Education.

**The American Anorexia/Bulimia Association**     No. 45

● http://members.aol.com/amanbu/index.html

Through the American Anorexia/Bulimia Association, a visitor can learn, and link to, information for those suffering from an eating disorder. Suggestions for families and friends of sufferers, details for professionals, and general information on eating disorders is also presented. Take the opportunity to browse a suggested newsgroup.

**Canadian Eating Disorders Sites**     No. 46

● http://www.stud.unit.no/studorg/ikstrh/ed/ed_cana.htm

Links-only site offering a list of eating disorder resources in Canada. Sources in various other countries are also provided.

**Eating Disorders Support Page**     No. 47

● http://www.geocities.com/SunsetStrip/3761/

Newsgroups, FAQs, and general information are the focus of this page. Look for links to additional resources.

## Making Your Own Connections

**Address/URL**

**Notes/Observations/
Site Description**

http://
_____

_____

_____

_____

http://
_____

_____

_____

_____

http://
_____

_____

_____

_____

http://
_____

_____

_____

_____

## Making Your Own Connections

**Address/URL**

**Notes/Observations/
Site Description**

http://
_____
_____
_____

http://
_____
_____
_____

http://
_____
_____
_____

http://
_____
_____
_____

# Ergogenic Aids ▬▬▬▬▬ 11

The term ergogenic implies "energy giving," but in reality, no product actually imparts this quality. Ergogenic aids include vitamin or mineral supplements, protein and amino acid supplements, steroids, and electrolyte pills. Athletes often take ergogenic supplements in the hope of gaining strength and improving performance. A variety of supplements make these claims, often based on a misunderstanding of nutrition and scientific concepts. The claims may sound plausible to an athlete, but they have no factual basis. Some of the ingredients may not have been tested, or there is little or no valid information available. Seldom do these products mention possible side effects.

Anabolic steroids are made naturally in the body. Men manufacture this hormone in the testes, and both men and women make it in the adrenal cortex. The steroids that some athletes take are synthetic versions that mix the growth stimulation of the adrenal steroids with the masculinizing effects of male hormones. The steroids produce accelerated muscle growth following physical activity. Although using these drugs increases strength and muscle size beyond what could be achieved by training alone, they do so at extreme health risks. These risks include aggression with hostility, mood swings, anxiety, and personality changes. (Source: "Steroids and Athletes: The Chemistry of Violence," *Addiction Letter,* May 1996.) Other side effects are changes in the heart and abdominal organs and increased risk of cancer, blood clots, AIDS from needle sharing, and damage to male and female reproductive systems.

Besides steroids, amino acid supplements or protein powders are popular among athletes. Generally, healthy athletes never need to add additional protein to their diet, since almost all Americans get more protein than is required. But, athletes take these supplements to build muscle. Because they tend to take high doses of amino acids, athletes may suffer harm. An excess of one or more amino acids can prevent absorption of others leading to a deficiency. In addition, the supplements are expensive.

Besides anabolic steroids and protein supplements, the vast majority of ergogenic aids designed for athletes are frauds. Although the placebo effect is at work, substances such as carnitine, bee pollen, and chromium picolinate are not what advertisers claim. Athletes make up a huge and favorable market for the supplement industry and will continue to be the target of aggressive marketing of ergogenic supplements. Despite the health risks, athletes believe in and use these products because of advertising, use by professional athletes and a strong desire to win at all costs. (Source: "Doped to Perfection," *Newsweek,* July 22, 1996.)

# Ergogenic Aids

What are some of the negative effects of anabolic steroids? Of amino acid supplements? • Why do athletes take these preparations?

## ⚫WebLinks

### Creatine: A Review of Its Uses in Sports                    No. 48
🌐 http://wwwnetstorage.com/hon/summary.html

This Web page was written by Dr. Clark from the University of Oxford. Dr. Clark provides a very thorough description of creatine and its role in athletics. There is a lengthy bibliography with additional research articles. This page is embedded in a commercial site that sells creatine monohydrate. But you do not need to buy anything . . . just read the excellent overview of creatine.

### Drug Education Page                                         No. 49
🌐 http://www.magic.mb.ca/~lampi/new_drugs.html

The Drug Education Page offers eclectic and thought-provoking material dealing with opinions on how to combat drug problems in society. Drugs discussed include marijuana, cocaine, steroids, and others. Links take visitors to related topics, including articles on the media, addiction, the war on drugs, and legality issues.

### Energy on the Run                                          No. 50
🌐 http://www.newsday.com/features/fcov0618.htm

This Web page is part of the *Newsday* electronic newspaper. This article provides a balanced perspective on the benefits of energy gels. This is *not* a research-based article; rather, it quotes athletes who have used energy gels and energy bars. As you read this article, decide whether or not you will contribute to the $10 million energy gel industry.

### International Study Group for Steroid Hormones             No. 51
🌐 http://www.elsevier.nl/estoc/publications/store/X/0039128X/

This is the official publication of the International Study Group for Steroid Hormones. Access to volumes of back issues and an editorial board is provided.

### Steroids                                                   No. 52
🌐 http://www.drugfreeamerica.org/steroids.html

From Partnership for a Drug-Free America, this site offers information and links on the negative effects of steroids. FAQs and tips on talking to a child about drugs are included.

## Making Your Own Connections

| Address/URL | Notes/Observations/Site Description |
|---|---|
| http://_____<br>_____<br>_____<br>_____ | |
| http://_____<br>_____<br>_____<br>_____ | |
| http://_____<br>_____<br>_____<br>_____ | |
| http://_____<br>_____<br>_____<br>_____ | |

# Ergogenic Aids

## *Making Your Own Connections*

| Address/URL | Notes/Observations/<br>Site Description |
|---|---|
| http:// | |
| http:// | |
| http:// | |
| http:// | |

# Ethnic Foods

Ethnic foods have become a part of the American diet. Recently, people have been flocking to Thai, Mexican, and Mediterranean-influenced restaurants and cooking these cuisines at home. Some ethnic diets are nutritious as well as tasty; others are high in fat and sodium. The diets of the people in the Mediterranean region—Italy, Spain, Portugal, France, Greece and North Africa—have been touted as healthful though high in fat. For instance, the diet in Greece contains over 40 percent of its calories from fat, mostly from olive oil and olives. In this country, we are urged to eat less than 30 percent of our calories as fat. Yet Greeks living in Greece enjoy one of the longest life expectancies in the world and die less often from heart disease. (Source: "The Virtues of the Mediterranean Diet: Illusion or Reality," *Chatelaine,* July 1996.) Heart disease death rates are also low among those living in Italy and Spain. Many questions, however, surround the Mediterranean diet. For instance, while heart disease rates may be low in these countries, the rate of strokes is almost double that of the United States. Although the relationship between diet and heart disease overall is strong, it is not clear which dietary component is responsible. Is it the olive oil or more seafood or the higher intake of fruits and vegetables?

Another interesting paradox is the Chinese diet. In China there is virtually no obesity even though people there eat approximately 20 percent more calories each day than do Americans. However, although the typical Chinese diet is higher in calories than the typical American diet, it is lower in fat. And the Chinese get considerably more exercise in their daily lives. Private car ownership is uncommon, and people walk or ride bicycles wherever they go. They also have much lower rates of serum cholesterol, heart disease, and certain cancers. Some Chinese dishes do have high levels of sodium, monosodium glutamate, and fat from deep frying. Deep frying in China, however, is done infrequently, as opposed to Chinese restaurants in this country. (Source: "Chinese Food O.K. For Most," *Family Circle,* February 1, 1996.)

Other popular cuisines in this country include Mexican and southern food. Mexican food can be either healthy or unhealthy. Good choices include beans, rice, tomato salsa, and cooked vegetables. Southern food includes healthful greens, okra, peas and beans, corn, sweet potatoes, cornbread and local fish. Unfortunately, many southern meals are very high in fat and sodium, including salt pork, bacon, fried chicken, biscuits and gravy, and spareribs.

# Ethnic Foods

 Why is the Mediterranean diet considered healthy? • How can the Chinese eat more calories and be thinner than Americans? • What are the drawbacks of a Chinese diet?

## ●WebLinks

### Gemini & Leo's Recipe Links                                    No. 53
● http://www.synapse.net/~gemini/recplink.htm

Comprehensive information and links feature recipes from magazines and personal collections. Access to various ethnic recipe sites, including Middle Eastern, barbeque, cajun, kosher, Medieval and Renaissance, is provided.

### Minority Health Resource Pocket Guide                         No. 54
● http://www.omhrc.gov/pocket/pocket.htm

Look for links to minority organizations, sources of health materials for minority populations, state minority health liaisons, and federal health information centers and clearing houses. Prepared by the Office of Minority Health Resource Center.

### Traditional Food, Health and Nutrition for Native Americans     No. 55
● http://indy4.fdl.cc.mn.us/~isk/food/foodmenu.html

Great site including dietary information for several Native American tribes in the U. S. Look for native and wild plant expertise, wild rice, secret native plant lore recipes and relevant food links.

### Yugoslav Cuisine                                               No. 56
● http://www.yugoslavia.com/Culture/HTML/food.html

Information is provided about the variety of cuisines in Yugoslavia, which result from ethnic and religious diversities coupled with the history, geography, and climate of the region. The site lists a large number of traditional foods and recipes.

## Making Your Own Connections

**Address/URL**

**Notes/Observations/
Site Description**

http://
_____
_____
_____

http://
_____
_____
_____

http://
_____
_____
_____

http://
_____
_____
_____

## Making Your Own Connections

| Address/URL | Notes/Observations/ Site Description |
|---|---|
| http:// | |
| http:// | |
| http:// | |
| http:// | |

# Food Additives 13

Although foodborne disease occurs mainly from bacteria and viruses, the safety of the food supply also depends on the level of additives and contaminants. Pesticide residues in food can occur from the direct spraying of crops or the consumption of pesticide-contaminated animal feed, which can show up in meat, eggs, or milk. The Environmental Protection Agency (EPA) has established tolerance levels for all pesticides used on food crops based on the maximum residue likely when agricultural chemicals are properly applied. Most consumers are unlikely to encounter high levels of pesticide residues, but there are concerns over food imported into the United States. Many banned chemicals are still used outside the U. S., and these pesticides show up on bananas and other imported foods. Some of these pesticides were banned in the U. S. because they were linked to cancer and birth defects. Other problems arise if consumers eat unwashed fruits and vegetables. Washing will remove most of the pesticide residues.

Consumers are also concerned about the effects of certain food additives. Additives are chemicals deliberately added to food to add color, flavor, nutritive value, or to maintain freshness. There are currently over 2,500 food additives in use, many actually improving the safety of the food supply. For instance, vitamin D is added to milk to improve its nutritional value. Other additives retard spoilage and prevent fats from becoming rancid. A large number of additives, however, are used purely for cosmetic purposes, and many of these have been linked to health problems. Food colors, sodium nitrite, monosodium glutamate (MSG), and sulfites are among the additives that have caused health concerns. (Source: "Analysis of Adverse Reactions to Monosodium Glutamate," *Journal of Nutrition*, 1995.) The majority of Americans show no ill effect from MSG or sulfites, but a minority of sensitive individuals, particularly asthmatics in the case of sulfites, have had severe reactions from eating these additives. Sulfites have been used for years to prevent discoloration and spoilage in a variety of foods and wines. After receiving more than 700 reports of adverse sulfite reactions, including several fatalities, the U. S. Food and Drug Administration (FDA) banned use of the additive on raw cut vegetables and fruits, a move directed mostly at salad bars, which were the source of most of the illnesses.

In response to the public's concerns, the FDA has approved only five new direct human food additives, including aspartame and olestra, since 1970. (Source: "Approval of Food Additives in the United States," *Food Technology*, March 1996.) Most of the additives currently in use are on the GRAS (Generally Regarded as Safe) list, a group of additives that are assumed to be safe though many have never been adequately tested.

# Food Additives

 What are the potential health effects of pesticide residues?  •
What are the concerns of eating imported fruits and vegetables?  •  What additive has been banned from salad bars?

# ●WebLinks

### Environmental Protection Agency                                No. 57
● http://www.epa.gov

User-friendly site from the Environmental Protection Agency (EPA) offers a
searchable database and comprehensive directory. Visitors can explore over a
dozen different aspects of this organization and can search for local offices by zip
code. Information concerning laws and regulations is provided.

### Food Additives                                                No. 58
● http://www.social.com/health/ific/food_additives/main.html

Links-only site from the International Food Information Council. Topics include
food colors, food additives, and U.S. Food and Drug Administration back-
grounds on Monsodium Glutamate (MSG).

### Food Additives and Premarket Approval                         No. 59
● http://vm.cfsan.fda.gov/~lrd/foodadd.html

Food additives and premarket approval are the focus of this page that provides
links to related topics. Worthwhile subjects covered: fat substitutes, food colors,
Monsodium Glutamate (MSG), sulfites, restrictions on U.S. Food and Drug Administration (FDA) approval, and others. This site is maintained by the FDA's
Center for Food Safety and Applied Nutrition.

### Pesticides                                                    No. 60
● http://ificinfo.health.org/index13.htm

A consumer's guide to pesticides, pesticides and food safety, pesticides Q&As,
and pesticides and children's health are some of the topics covered at this site
maintained by the International Food Information Council. Brochures, reviews,
and food insight reports are also included. Links provided.

### Pesticides, Metals & Industrial Chemicals                     No. 61
● http://vm.cfsan.fda.gov/~lrd/pestadd.html

From the Center for Food Safety and Applied Nutrition of the U.S. Food and
Drug Administration, this reliable site offers links to reports on pesticides in
foods, a glossary of pesticide chemicals, and related reports discussing both general and technical information. Links connect to pages providing details on common metal and chemical food concerns and regulatory data.

## Making Your Own Connections

| Address/URL | Notes/Observations/ Site Description |
|---|---|
| http:// _____ _____ _____ _____ | |
| http:// _____ _____ _____ _____ | |
| http:// _____ _____ _____ _____ | |
| http:// _____ _____ _____ _____ | |

## Making Your Own Connections

**Address/URL**

**Notes/Observations/
Site Description**

http://

_____

_____

_____

http://

_____

_____

_____

http://

_____

_____

_____

http://

_____

_____

_____

# Food Allergies 14

Food allergy is thought to be a common occurrence among children and adults. In actuality, less than eight percent of children and two percent of adults suffer from true food allergies. (Source: "Mechanisms of Food Allergy," *Annual Review of Nutrition*, Volume 16, 1996.) A true food allergy occurs when the protein in food enters body tissues. Some of these proteins are not digested but enter the bloodstream whole. Once they are inside the bloodstream, the body's immune system releases defensive agents known as antibodies that cause allergic responses. These responses include cramping, bloating, nausea, diarrhea or vomiting, hives, swelling, rashes, or runny nose. A severe and potentially fatal reaction is anaphylactic shock.

Unfortunately, it is not always easy to determine what foods cause these symptoms. Reactions to food can occur within minutes or up to 24 hours after eating. Many people are allergic to one food only, although some are allergic to many. About three-quarters of allergic reactions are caused by three foods: milk, eggs, and peanuts. The life-threatening reaction of anaphylactic shock most often is the result of eating shellfish, fish, nuts, or peanuts. (Source: "Family Allergies? Keep Nuts Away From Baby," *Science News*, May 4, 1996.) The treatment for food allergies is to avoid the offending food or foods. Fortunately, many people outgrow food allergies.

Tests to diagnose food allergies are often expensive and time consuming. Many people or their physicians may diagnose food allergies without adequately testing. Parents whose child(ren) have any kind of discomfort following eating may determine that an allergy is responsible when in fact the cause may be something else entirely. Many people believe they have an allergy to milk if they experience discomfort after drinking it. What most of these people are probably experiencing is the more common lactose intolerance, not milk allergy. Lactose intolerance is not related to milk protein but to the carbohydrate in milk known as lactose. Some children and adults lose the ability to produce the enzyme necessary to digest lactose. After drinking milk, these individuals experience diarrhea, nausea, and gas. Many lactose intolerant adults and children can tolerate small amounts of milk at a time, while others are extremely sensitive. To avoid the symptoms, specially treated milk can be used. Other dairy products that are low in lactose include yogurt or aged cheese. People with true milk allergies often cannot tolerate cheese or yogurt either and need to avoid these foods. (Source: "Lactose Intolerance," *Harvard Women's Health Watch*, October 1996.)

# Food Allergies

**?** Which foods are most likely to cause allergic reactions? •
What is the difference between milk allergy and lactose intolerance? • What are some of the problems in diagnosing a
food allergy? • What are some of the common symptoms associated
with food allergies? • How common are food allergies among
adults? Among children? • What is the most severe type of food
reaction?

## ●WebLinks

### Allergy, Asthma & Immunology Online　　　No. 62
● http://allergy.mcg.edu/Advice/foods.html

Text only Q&As about food allergies, including origins, symptoms, and testing.
Statistics and links to help visitors find local allergists are incorporated. Valu-
able information is presented concisely by the American College of Allergy,
Asthma and Immunology.

### Allergy Internet Resources　　　No. 63
● http://www.io.com/~kinnaman/allabc.html

Abundant links offer details on all types of allergies, asthma, testing, access to
health care, and a keyword search engine. Learn about electronic mailing lists
and USENET Newsgroups or search for local doctors.

### Doctor's Guide to Allergies　　　No. 64
● http://www.pslgroup.com/ALLERGIES.HTM

Broad site provides extensive array of links to issues in the news, medical news
and alerts, allergy information, discussion groups, newsgroups, and related
sites. Sign up for notification of additions or changes to the list.

### Food Allergy and Intolerances　　　No. 65
● http://www.niaid.nih.gov/publications/food/full.htm

From the National Institute of Allergy and Infectious Diseases of the National
Institutes of Health, text describes food allergy symptoms and how allergic reactions work. Q&As are also provided.

### The Food Allergy Network　　　No. 66
● http://www.foodallergy.org

Look for reliable data on product alerts, facts and fiction about food allergies,
answers to common questions, and daily tips. Visitors can link to consumer
information, professional information, and related reports.

## Making Your Own Connections

| Address/URL | Notes/Observations/ Site Description |
| --- | --- |
| http:// | |
| http:// | |
| http:// | |
| http:// | |

## Making Your Own Connections

**Address/URL**

**Notes/Observations/
Site Description**

http://
_____
_____
_____

http://
_____
_____
_____

http://
_____
_____
_____

http://
_____
_____
_____

# Food Composition 15

Eating a healthy diet is easy, in theory. All one has to do is eat a variety of foods that supplies necessary amounts of the essential nutrients, calories, and fiber without an excess of calories, fat, salt, or sugar. Although some people manage to eat foods that meet their needs, many of us do not as evidenced by the number of overweight and malnourished individuals in this country. (Source: "Healthy People 2000 at Mid Decade," *JAMA,* Volume 273, 1995.) People's diets are inadequate for a variety of reasons: time, money, food preferences, indifference, and lack of knowledge. Many people still believe, for instance, that bread and potatoes are fattening and avoid these foods. Others skip meals in an effort to lose weight. There are many resources available to help people eat a healthy diet, but not everyone is aware of them or how they are used. Some of these resources include food labels and tables of food composition.

On all food labels there must be a list of ingredients in order of descending weight and daily values. Labels must list standard serving size, number of servings per package, total calories per serving, calories from fat per serving, and total fat grams, with a breakdown of saturated fat, total cholesterol, sodium, carbohydrates, fiber, sugars and protein, vitamins A and C, calcium and iron. A quick glance at a package label will indicate if the food is nutrient dense, supplying a lot of nutrients in relation to the total calories. (Source: "Food Label Makes Good Eating Easier," *FDA Consumer,* September 1995.) For a sample food label and instructions on how to read it, turn to Appendix A.

Tables of food composition can help supply the knowledge needed to eat a healthy diet. These tables list hundreds, and sometimes thousands, of foods, their calorie content, and nutritional values. They are available in government documents, reports, scientific journals, industry analyses, text books, software, and online. (Source: "Composition of Food: Agriculture Handbook No. 8" *USDA,* 1995.) Many chain restaurants also evaluate their menu offerings and produce nutritional information on their products.

Being aware of and eating nutrient-dense foods allows most people to meet their nutrition needs without gaining weight. Having valid sources of information about restaurant and home-cooked food can help in the process of planning and eating a healthier diet.

# Food Composition

| ? | What does the term nutrient dense mean? • What information is on a food label? • What information is on a table of food composition? • What are some sources of tables of food composition? |

## ●WebLinks

### Center for Science in the Public Interest     No. 67
🌐 http://www.cspinet.org/

The Center for Science in the Public Interest is a nonprofit education and advocacy organization that focuses on improving the safety and nutritional quality of our food supply and on reducing the health problems caused by alcohol. This agency also evaluates the nutritional composition of fast foods, movie popcorn, and chain restaurants. Good links to related sites.

### Fast Food Facts—Interactive Food Finder     No. 68
🌐 http://www.olen.com/food/

This interactive site from Olen Publishing Company provides various options for identifying nutrient information on foods at many of the popular fast food restaurants. It can also create a menu based on a specific nutritional profile. This information can help people make healthful choices at fast food restaurants. Based on the book *Fast Food Facts* by the Minnesota Attorney General's office.

### Nutrient Data Laboratory     No. 69
🌐 http://www.nal.usda.gov/fnic/foodcomp/

Maintained by the U.S. Department of Agriculture's Research Service's Nutrient Data Laboratory, visitors can research food items in a nutrition database, understand food composition products, browse FAQs, and examine a glossary of terms. Data on Chinese and Swiss foods are included. Links provided.

### Nutrient Database     No. 70
🌐 http://www.nutribase.com

Complete, informative site offers interactive online database that provides nutrient details on 19,344 food items (primarily U.S. Department of Agriculture SR 10 data) and 3,160 menu items from 71 chain restaurants. Easily navigated, visitors can search for, view, and rank foods by name. Links to the nutrition database contain information on software, food manufacturers, news, and feedback. Also included are calculators to compute calorie requirements and weight loss and charts indicating desirable weight and body fat.

## Making Your Own Connections

| Address/URL | Notes/Observations/ Site Description |
|---|---|
| http:// | |
| http:// | |
| http:// | |
| http:// | |

## Making Your Own Connections

| Address/URL | Notes/Observations/ Site Description |
|---|---|
| http:// _____ _____ _____ _____ | |
| http:// _____ _____ _____ _____ | |
| http:// _____ _____ _____ _____ | |
| http:// _____ _____ _____ _____ | |

# Food Guide Pyramid 16
## & Dietary Guidelines

In the past, Americans were taught to eat from the basic seven foods that became the Four Food Group Plan: milk, meat, fruits and vegetables, and grains. Today the message is to eat from five groups: grains, fruits and vegetables, milk, protein, and fats and oils. These groups are represented by the Food Guide Pyramid. The pyramid shape of the food guide has a broad base of grains at the bottom and conveys the idea that we should be eating more grain foods than anything else. Serving sizes are given as a range. For instance, the number of grain servings for adults is from six to eleven per day. After grains, the next level of the pyramid is made up of fruits and vegetables. Milk and animals foods are higher up, followed by fats, oils, and sweets at the point of the pyramid. The food pyramid is a simple tool that graphically shows that it is preferable to eat more grains and fruits and vegetables than meat or milk. Although meat and milk are rich in nutrients such as protein, vitamins, and minerals, they can be high in fat and calories and low in fiber. (Source: "Protein Pitfalls," *American Fitness,* July/August 1996.)

The pyramid can be useful in planning a healthy diet, but it does have some drawbacks. It doesn't emphasize foods low in calories, and a person may select the correct number of servings from each food group yet make choices within the group that do not supply adequate nutrients. For example, eating only apples for the fruit group and only iceberg lettuce for the vegetables would put the person at risk for vitamin C deficiency.

The food pyramid, however, can be a valuable tool in quickly assessing the adequacy of the diet. Another tool is the Dietary Guidelines for Americans. The guidelines supply a general list of recommendations regarding a healthy diet. (Source: "Dietary Guidelines for Americans," *USDA, Home and Garden Bulletin,* No. 232, 1995.)

The first recommendation is to eat a variety of foods, which can prevent nutritional deficiencies. Other recommendations include eating a diet with plenty of grain products, vegetables, and fruits. Unlike the pyramid, the Dietary Guidelines provide general advice and make no specific serving size recommendations. The Dietary Guidelines, unlike the pyramid, recommend that we balance the food we eat with enough physical activity to maintain or achieve ideal body weight.

# Food Guide Pyramid & Dietary Guidelines

**?** What foods should be eaten in the greatest quantity according to the food pyramid? • Which foods should be eaten only occasionally? • What are some of the drawbacks of using the food pyramid?

## ●Web*Links*

### Dietary Guidelines for Americans      No. 71
● http://www.nal.usda.gov/fnic/dga/

This straightforward page from the U.S. Department of Agriculture provides links to the 1995 and 1990 editions of Dietary Guidelines for Americans and a link to the 1995 Report of the Dietary Guidelines Advisory Committee on the Dietary Guidelines for Americans. Further links help streamline searches.

### Food Guide Pyramid Information      No. 72
● http://www.nal.usda.gov/fnic/Fpyr/pyramid.html

This links-only site offers an interactive food guide pyramid. A visitor can gain detailed information by clicking on topics of interest. Available software is also described.

### Health Fax Heart-Healthy Diet      No. 73
● http://www.smtmoves.com/healthfax/hdiet.html

This site offers explanations of how your diet can affect your heart. From this Web page, you will learn how to increase antioxidants and reduce fat and cholesterol in your diet.

### Nutrition and Your Health: Dietary Guidelines for Americans      No. 74
● http://vm.cfsan.fda.gov/~dms/nutguide.html

This extensive text-only site explains the food pyramid and dietary guidelines for Americans. It is maintained by the U.S. Food and Drug Administration's Center for Food Safety and Applied Nutrition.

# Food Guide Pyramid & Dietary Guidelines

## Making Your Own Connections

| Address/URL | Notes/Observations/ Site Description |
|---|---|
| http://  _____ _____ _____ | |
| http://  _____ _____ _____ | |
| http://  _____ _____ _____ | |
| http://  _____ _____ _____ | |

# Food Guide Pyramid & Dietary Guidelines

## Making Your Own Connections

Address/URL

Notes/Observations/
Site Description

http://

_____

_____

_____

http://

_____

_____

_____

http://

_____

_____

_____

http://

_____

_____

_____

# Food Safety

Early in this century, contaminated food, milk and water were responsible for many large outbreaks of diseases including diphtheria, typhoid fever, and other infections. Since that time, safe water and milk have become available, but the greatest health risk comes from food contaminated from bacteria and other microbes.

Up to one-half of the cases of diarrhea in the U.S. are caused by foodborne organisms. Food poisoning can also produce vomiting, fever, cramps, and seizures. The contamination of food is thought to be responsible for at least 9,000 deaths each year. The risk of foodborne illness is high because of recent changes in our lifestyle, including eating away from home more often, eating more imported foods, and the increase in the number of vulnerable people, such as the elderly. Still another cause of increased foodborne diseases is improved diagnosis and reporting. (Source: "Are Foodborne Bacteria Becoming More Deadly?" *Health,* October 1996.)

To keep food safe, it should be thoroughly cooked, kept either cold or hot, stored and reheated carefully, and protected from insects and rodents. In addition, raw food, especially animal foods, should be separated from cooked food to avoid contamination.

In the short term, microbial food poisoning is our greatest concern. In the long term, there are other risks, including additives, pesticides, and genetically engineered foods. Genetically engineered food is created by removing the genetic material from one organism and inserting it into another. Certain characteristics of plants and animals are passed on. The new organism, known as a transgenic, can be produced less expensively and more nutritionally. Currently, limited tests have been conducted to find out the impact of transgenic foods on humans. A study published in the *New England Journal of Medicine* has shown that some genetically engineered food has the potential to cause allergic reactions. (Source: "Trying to Get Labels on Genetically Engineered Food," *New York Times,* May 21, 1997.) In a study at the University of Nebraska, a gene from a Brazil nut was inserted into a soybean. The genetically altered soybean was tested on people who had a known allergy to Brazil nuts. It was found that they had a similar allergic reaction to the Brazil nut-modified soybeans but not to the original soybean. Without labels identifying the soybean as genetically modified, allergic individuals run the risk of a reaction which could be severe or even fatal. (Source: "Food Scare," *New Scientist,* March 16, 1996.)

# Food Safety

 Why has food been genetically altered? • In the short term, what is the greatest food risk? • Why has food poisoning been increasing lately?

## ●WebLinks

### Center for Food Safety and Applied Nutrition                   No. 75
● http://www.mothernature.com/links.htm

Multiple links to U. S. Food and Drug Administration sites and other government and non-government food safety and nutrition sites are found here. Hot keys allow visitors to perform keyword searches, purchase health foods online, or obtain a catalog.

### Food Safety Home Page                   No. 76
● http://home.earthlink.net/~zinkd/index.html

This page is a resource for the causes and preventions of foodborne illnesses. Look for information on the microbes that cause foodborne diseases, factual information on current food safety issues, and details on foodborne illness outbreaks, including Bovine Spongiform Encephalopathy (Mad Cow Disease). Links to related food safety sites including government, university, and industry pages.

### Institute of Food Technologists                   No. 77
● http://www.ift.org/

Presented by the Institute of Food Technologists, visitors can get current news on food safety, search tables of contents from selected journals, and discover more about educational and career opportunities. Links provide access to daily news, commodity updates, and details on the institute.

### National Center for Food Safety & Technology (NCFST)                   No. 78
● http://www.iit.edu/~ncfs/

NCFST is a consortium organized to address the complex issues raised by emerging food technologies. It is through this organization that academia, industry, and government come together to pool their resources and work together to ensure continued safety and quality of the nation's food supply. This site offers current events, research topics, further resources, and educational programs in food safety. Links to related sites are available.

## Making Your Own Connections

**Address/URL**

**Notes/Observations/
Site Description**

http://
_____

_____

_____

_____

http://
_____

_____

_____

_____

http://
_____

_____

_____

_____

http://
_____

_____

_____

_____

## Making Your Own Connections

| Address/URL | Notes/Observations/ Site Description |
|---|---|
| http:// | |
| http:// | |
| http:// | |
| http:// | |

# HIV/AIDS & Nutrition ▬▬▬▬ 18

Acquired immune deficiency disease (AIDS) is caused by the human immunodeficiency virus (HIV), which attacks and destroys cells that are integral to the body's immune system. Without a healthy immune system, an HIV-infected person becomes vulnerable to opportunistic infections, including pneumonia and foodborne diseases. Adequate nutrition, while not a cure, can generally improve the quality, and possibly the quantity, of life. A person with AIDS who is well nourished can often remain healthy and independent longer than if nutrition had not been optimal. (Source: "AIDS Update," *Men's Health*, November 1996.)

There are two primary nutritional concerns regarding people with AIDS: wasting and food safety. Severe malnutrition with wasting of lean body tissue (protein energy malnutrition) is common in people with AIDS. It appears to be related to inadequate food intake, poor nutrient absorption, losses of fluids and nutrients associated with persistent diarrhea, medication reactions, and increased nutritional requirements. Even before an HIV-positive person is diagnosed with AIDS, the loss of lean body mass may occur, so attention to eating healthy may delay the onset of AIDS. (Source: "Research in AIDS Wasting and Nutrition Presented," *AIDS Weekly Plus*, July 29, 1996.)

Protein energy malnutrition is especially destructive to various immune-system organs and tissues. The digestive system is especially active in this regard. The mucous membranes of this system contain active immune tissues. During protein energy malnutrition, these cells dwindle in both number and size, opening the body to infection.

Related to wasting and malnutrition, people with AIDS often have difficulty eating. They may have mouth sores, trouble swallowing, or lack of appetite. Small, frequent meals, vitamin and mineral pills, and liquid meal supplements may help prevent weight loss. Liquid supplements are useful because they are also easy to swallow. (Source: "Nutritional Issues," *AIDS Weekly Plus*, November 11, 1996.)

A second major concern among HIV positive persons is food safety. Episodes of food poisoning cause illness in up to one-third of the U. S. population each year. Foodborne illness can be caused directly by microorganisms or by toxins produced by bacteria in the digestive tract. For most people, the symptoms are relatively mild and last no more than a few days. For individuals who are malnourished, who are HIV positive, or suffer from AIDS, these disturbances can be very serious and possibly fatal. These people need to pay particular attention to food safety, making sure their food is well cooked, stored properly, and clean.

# HIV/AIDS & Nutrition

**?** What are the two primary nutritional concerns among AIDS patients? • Why do AIDS patients often suffer from wasting syndrome? • What are some dietary recommendations for AIDS patients?

## ●Web*Links*

### The Body: An AIDS and HIV Information Resource                        No. 79
● http://www.thebody.com/cgi/treatans.html

This comprehensive site presented by three physicians provides articles and answers to questions about treatments, including drug therapy, alternative treatments, nutrition, and mental health issues related to HIV and AIDS. Visitors can post additional questions for response. Links to experts and government agencies and a search engine are furnished.

### Gay Men's Health Center                        No. 80
● http://www.gmhc.org/living/living.html

The Gay Men's Health Center of New York maintains this page that features topics of interest to persons who are HIV positive or who are living with AIDS. Subjects covered include nutrition, alcohol and drugs, medical care and treatment, support groups, financial and legal concerns, insurance, and emergency services. A survey is provided for visitors who wish to participate.

### HIVnALIVE                        No. 81
● http://www.hivnalive.org

Although challenging, this site presents data on improving the quality of life for a person who is HIV positive or living with AIDS. Links provide access to information on nutrition, other organizations and additional resources. Maintained by HIVnALIVE.

### Medpatients Network                        No. 82
● http://www.medpatients.com/aids.htm

Look for current news on AIDS, a fact sheet, and details of AIDS research. A short list of links also provides access to AEGIS, AIDSCAP, a discussion group, and a resource list.

### National Food Safety Database: Food Safety for At-Risk Groups                        No. 83
● http://www.foodsafety.org/aidhome.htm

This section of the National Food Safety Database is dedicated to persons most susceptible to foodborne illnesses. Link to related sites on eating defensively, vulnerable individuals and increased risk of foodborne illness, and safe food for vulnerable people.

## Making Your Own Connections

| Address/URL | Notes/Observations/ Site Description |
|---|---|
| http://  _____  _____  _____  _____ | |
| http://  _____  _____  _____  _____ | |
| http://  _____  _____  _____  _____ | |
| http://  _____  _____  _____  _____ | |

## Making Your Own Connections

| Address/URL | Notes/Observations/ Site Description |
|---|---|
| http:// | |
| http:// | |
| http:// | |
| http:// | |

# Lactation and Infant Feeding ■ 19

National efforts to promote breastfeeding have met with some success, but less than 20 percent of infants in this country are breastfed for more than one or two months. There are numerous advantages of extended breastfeeding, including nutritional, psychological, economic, and immunological. Human milk provides optimal nutrition to infants with its appropriate balance of nutrients and digestibility. Minerals in breast milk are perfectly balanced, while the fat in human milk promotes optimal development of the central nervous system. Breastfeeding, in addition to offering infants optimal nutrition, also supplies babies with antibodies to protect against disease. In studies performed in both industrialized and non-industrialized countries, breastfed babies have been reported to have significantly fewer gastrointestinal illnesses, respiratory problems, allergies, and ear infections. (Source: "Breastfeeding and Infant Mortality," *International Family Planning Perspectives,* September 1996.)

Mothers also benefit from breastfeeding. Studies have shown women who breastfeed their children are more likely to lose the weight they gained during pregnancy. Breastfeeding may also offer some protection against breast cancer. (Source: "Improved Maternal Health and Infant Survival," *Women's Health Weekly,* January 22, 1996.) In addition, it is considerably less expensive to breastfeed than to purchase formula and bottles.

With all the benefits to breastfeeding, why do so few women continue after the first few months? Overall, slightly less than 60 percent of women leave the hospital breastfeeding. The highest incidence of women who nurse their babies are older than 30 years, college educated, and in higher income groups. (Source: "Position of the American Dietetic Association: Promotion of Breast-Feeding," *Journal of the American Dietetics Association,* June 1997.) While there has been an increase among some high risk groups, less than 10 percent of low income babies are being breastfed.

Barriers to breastfeeding include social and cultural factors, inadequate training of physicians and other providers, shorter hospital stays, and short maternity leaves from work. The marketing of infant formulas, which includes free samples in hospital discharge packages, may promote the use of these products over breastfeeding.

Although few women are physically unable to breastfeed, about 40 percent begin feeding their babies formula or discontinue breastfeeding after one or two months. Many of the well-recognized benefits of breastfeeding are significantly greater with exclusive breast feeding for at least four months.

# Lactation and Infant Feeding

**?** What are the advantages of breastfeeding for infants? For mothers? • Why do so few low income women breast feed? • Should hospitals continue to distribute baby formula to new mothers?

## ●Web*Links*

### Breastfeeding Advocacy Page                                          No. 84
● http://www.clark.net/pub/activist/bfpage/bfpage.html

This page is dedicated to providing education on, and promoting, breastfeeding. An array of links presents information on why breastfeeding is important, the dangers associated with formula feeding, and a discussion of why breastfeeding rates are low. Narratives are interspersed with links to additional sites or other views.

### Breastfeeding Information on the Web                                  No. 85
● http://www.efn.org/~djz/birth/breastfeeding/html

Search the Online Birth Center for articles, books, videos, products, and organizations that support breastfeeding, or review the nursing tips provided. Newsgroups and other resources are available. Useful links give access to related pages.

### Infant Feeding Action Coalition (INFACT) Canada                       No. 86
● http://www.io.org/~infacto

INFACT is a nonprofit, voluntary organization that promotes maternal and infant health by promoting breastfeeding and fostering appropriate mother and infant nutrition. This site explains the problems caused by declines in breastfeeding.

### Institute of Reproductive Health                                      No. 87
● http://www.irh.org

The Breastfeeding and Maternal and Child Health Division of the Institute for Reproductive Health provides answers to FAQs, access to a bookstore, and links to domestic and international resources on breastfeeding.

### La Leche League                                                       No. 88
● http://www.lalecheleague.org/

La Leche League International is an international, nonprofit organization dedicated to providing encouragement to women who wish to breastfeed. This site contains a broad range of links that provides access to educational, informational and support programs offered by the league. An overview and history of La Leche, information on services provided to women and health care professionals, answers to FAQs, and an opportunity to search for a local La Leche leader are included.

### World Alliance for Breast Feeding Action                             No. 89
● http://bbs.elogica.com.br/waba/

International links to information about breastfeeding are featured at this site. Other topics include a description of the World Alliance for Breast Feeding Action, the Lactational Amenorrhea Method (LAM) page, and breastfeeding resources.

# Lactation and Infant Feeding

## Making Your Own Connections

Address/URL

Notes/Observations/
Site Description

http://

_____

_____

_____

http://

_____

_____

_____

http://

_____

_____

_____

http://

_____

_____

_____

# Lactation and Infant Feeding

## Making Your Own Connections

| Address/URL | Notes/Observations/ Site Description |
|---|---|
| http://_____ _____ _____ _____ | |
| http://_____ _____ _____ _____ | |
| http://_____ _____ _____ _____ | |
| http://_____ _____ _____ _____ | |

Until recently, most commercial weight loss programs directed their marketing efforts towards women. The weight loss industry, which has been growing in total revenue by more than 10 percent a year, aims its products and services at the large number of overweight Americans. But the 1990s has been a period of slower growth, so the companies are looking to a new market: men. Major weight loss programs have begun to target men in their ads and consider men to be their prime growth area. (Source: "Lean for Life," *Men's Health,* July/August 1996.)

The diet companies' growth has paralleled the rise in obesity rates in this country, which have gone from one quarter of the population to 33 percent today. Although both men and women are affected, most participants in weight reduction programs are women for a variety of social and cultural reasons. Men, however, are increasingly becoming concerned about their weight for appearance and health reasons, and the diet industry is hoping to lure more men into weight loss programs.

Health concerns such as heart disease and certain cancers are closely linked to weight and overall nutrition. The leading cause of death among men in this country is heart disease, which is related to obesity and a diet high in fats, especially saturated fats. Men are at risk for heart disease earlier in life than women. Eating less total fat, more dietary fiber, and less animal foods is correlated to a lowered rate of heart disease. Animal foods are also linked to certain cancers, including colon and prostate. Prostate cancer will affect one in five men in North America. Studies have found that diets low in animal foods, overall calories and saturated fats in particular can help reduce the risk of prostate cancer. (Source: "Fat Chance," *Men's Health,* October 1996.) In addition to reducing fats and calories, a recent study has found that tomato-based foods may help lower the risk of prostate cancer. A group of over 47,000 men were asked about their intake of tomato products, including sauce, pizza, juice, and fresh and cooked tomatoes. The study, which was part of the Health Professionals Follow-up Study, found that tomatoes and foods made with tomatoes were significantly associated with lower prostate cancer risk. Researchers note that these foods are high in the naturally occurring plant chemical lycopene, which appears to reduce cancer risk. (Source: "Intake of Carotenoids and Retinol in Relation to Risk of Prostate Cancer," *Journal of the National Cancer Institute,* December 6, 1995.)

# Men's Nutrition

**?** What foods should be eaten to reduce the risk of prostate cancer? • Why are men being targeted by weight reduction companies? • What is the leading cause of death among men in this country? • What foods are linked to heart disease? • What naturally-occurring chemical in tomatoes is linked to a reduced risk of heart disease?

## ●WebLinks

### Eating Disorders in Males                    No. 90
● http://www.mhsource.com/edu/psytimes/p950942.html

For those who think eating disorders is a female-only condition, this site dispels that myth. Look for fact sheet on eating disorders among men maintained by Mental Health Infosource.

### Men's Health Magazine                    No. 91
● http://www.menshealth.com/index.html

Maintained by Men's Health Magazine, this site provides interesting and comprehensive details on topics of interest to men. Look for weekly tips, an opportunity to ask questions about men's health, and information related to nutrition and fitness. Links provide answers to FAQs, events, resources, the current month's issue, health Q&As, sex Q&As, letters to the editor, and other useful information.

### Men's Nutrition Page                    No. 92
● http://www.healthtouch.com/level1/leaflets/101529/101530.htm

Links-only site offers information on nutrition and weight control, sports nutrition, and nutrition and the elderly. This site is maintained by Healthtouch Online.

### Prostate Cancer                    No. 93
● http://www.comed.com/Prostate/index.html

Prostate cancer has been linked to a diet high in saturated fat. This award-winning site of the CoMed Communications Internet Health Forum offers information on the disease, including diagnosis, treatment, support, and prevention. Hot keys lead to the latest information and statistics.

## Making Your Own Connections

Address/URL

Notes/Observations/
Site Description

http://
_____
_____
_____

http://
_____
_____
_____

http://
_____
_____
_____

http://
_____
_____
_____

## Making Your Own Connections

| Address/URL | Notes/Observations/ Site Description |
|---|---|
| http:// | |
| http:// | |
| http:// | |
| http:// | |

# Nutrients (Carbohydrates, Fats & Protein) 21

Vital components in food are known as nutrients. The nutrients in foods are water, carbohydrate, fat, protein, vitamins, and minerals. Of these six, carbohydrates, protein, and fat supply calories, or energy, to the body. Protein also provides the body with the raw material necessary to build and repair cells.

Most Americans get more than enough protein in their diets. Although protein is an important part of the diet, too much is unnecessary and, for some individuals, may be harmful. A lot of the protein we eat is found in high fat foods such as meat or cheese. In fact, meat is the largest source of saturated fat in the average American's diet. (Source: "Protein Pitfalls," *American Fitness*, July/August 1996.) Meat is also devoid of dietary fiber, mostly indigestible roughage that aids in digestion and may help prevent cancer and heart disease. Most of us get all the protein we need, but many Americans get about half of the recommended fiber. Fiber is found only in fruits, vegetables, whole grains, nuts and seeds. (Source: "Fiber: Your Intestine's Best Friend," *Executive Health's Good Health Report*, January 1997.)

Although protein can be used by the body as a source of energy, the most efficient energy is supplied by carbohydrates and fats. Carbohydrates, or sugars and starches, offer the body well-utilized energy. Carbohydrate foods, which are wrongly accused of being fattening, contain no more calories ounce per ounce than lean protein. Fat, on the other hand, supplies over twice the calories as carbohydrates. Starchy foods, or complex carbohydrates, also supply the body with valuable nutrients. For instance, whole grains, dried beans (legumes), and vegetables are not only excellent sources of fiber, these foods also contain B vitamins, minerals, and are mostly low in fat. Refined sugars, on the other hand, offer the body only calories. A tablespoon of sugar contains 50 calories and no other nutrients. Fruits, which contain natural sugars, are different nutritionally from refined sugars. Fruits supply the body with fiber, vitamins, and minerals.

The best way to supply the nutrients the body needs is by eating a varied diet high in whole grains, fruits, vegetables, and a moderate amount of lean protein foods. The lowest fat protein foods include very lean meats, skinless chicken breast, skim milk, egg whites, and dried beans.

# Nutrients (Carbohydrates, Fats & Protein)

 Which foods are good sources of complex carbohydrates?
- What nutrient may be deficient from the American diet?
- Which nutrient contains the most calories?

## ❂WebLinks

### Carbohydrates: Fueling Up                                    No. 94
❂ http://ificinfo.health.org/insight/carbo.htm

The International Food Information Council (IFIC) presents this text-only guide to carbohydrates. Visitors can browse a glossary or search through text for desired material. Related documents are available by returning to IFIC's homepage.

### Consumer's Guide to Fats                                    No. 95
❂ http://www.fda.gov/opacom/catalog/conguide.html

A Consumer's Guide to Fats by Eleanor Mayfield is provided by the U. S. Food and Drug Administration. This narrative contains some important issues concerning fats.

### Fat: How Much is Too Much?                                  No. 96
❂ http://h-devil-www.mc.duke.edu/h-devil/nutrit/fat.htm

This text-only page presents a fact sheet on fats and includes a chart on fat grams in common foods. The site is provided by Duke University and questions may be posed through the Healthy Devil Online homepage.

### Sweeteners                                                  No. 97
❂ http://ificinfo.health.org/index8.htm

Links-only source of information on sugars and health, fructose, and aspartame. The International Food Information Council supplies reviews, Q&As, and food insight reports.

### Upbeat on Fiber                                             No. 98
❂ http://ificinfo.health.org/insight/upfiber.htm

Look for a text-only overview of fiber from the International Food Information Council. A chart with sources of several types of fiber is included.

# Nutrients (Carbohydrates, Fats & Proteins)

## Making Your Own Connections

| Address/URL | Notes/Observations/ Site Description |
|---|---|
| http:// _____ _____ _____ _____ | |
| http:// _____ _____ _____ _____ | |
| http:// _____ _____ _____ _____ | |
| http:// _____ _____ _____ _____ | |

# Nutrients (Carbohydrates, Fats & Proteins)

## Making Your Own Connections

| Address/URL | Notes/Observations/ Site Description |
|---|---|
| http:// | |
| http:// | |
| http:// | |
| http:// | |

# Nutrition and Alcohol 22

Several recent studies have shown that teetolers have a greater risk of developing heart problems than moderate drinkers and alcohol may be a risk factor for breast cancer. Findings about the relationship between alcohol and health have been conflicting, to say the least. A study published in the *Archives of Internal Medicine* found that men who had two to six alcoholic drinks per week had the lowest risk of death, while men who had two or more drinks per day had the highest risk of death. (Source: "Prospective Study of Moderate Alcohol Consumption and Mortality in U.S. Male Physicians," January 13, 1997.) A study reported in the *Tufts University Diet & Nutrition Letter* found that three to five drinks a day are associated with the greatest longevity for men and women! (Source: August 1995.)

How does alcohol affect longevity? Alcohol appears to help prevent blood clots that could block the flow of blood to the heart. It also raises HDL cholesterol (the "good" cholesterol), which lowers the risk of heart disease. Although alcohol increases HDL levels, exercising and losing excess weight raises them even more. For women, the relationship between alcohol and breast cancer and fetal alcohol syndrome seems to negate any heart health benefits.

Researchers agree on two issues: Moderate drinking is roughly defined as no more than two drinks per day for men and one drink per day for women, and no one should take up drinking for the express purpose of reducing their heart disease risk. The potential for alcohol abuse, health problems, and alcohol-related car accidents is too strong. In addition to these problems, alcohol contains calories. Most beer, wines, or other alcoholic drinks contain at least 100 calories. Alcohol also can affect nutritional status. Excessive drinking can deplete the body of essential nutrients like B vitamins. It also can affect appetite and digestion. Excessive drinking is a risk factor for cirrhosis of the liver, certain cancers, brain damage, and stroke.

Despite these disadvantages, alcohol does appear to offer heart-health benefits. Although alcoholic beverage labels carry warnings that state that drinking is harmful, especially for pregnant women and drivers, two free-market public-interest groups are suing the government to allow alcohol labels to carry information about potential health *benefits*. (Source: "Drink to Your Heart's Content?" *Insight*, March 3, 1997.) Plus, the U.S. Department of Agriculture has changed its *Dietary Guidelines for Americans* to state that "Current evidence suggests that moderate drinking is associated with a lower risk of coronary heart disease in some individuals."

# Nutrition and Alcohol

**?** Do you know what constitutes moderate drinking? • Why should recommendations differ for men and women? • How does alcohol affect nutritional status? • Should warning labels on alcoholic beverages be adjusted to suggest that drinking has health advantages?

## ⊗WebLinks

### Alcohol and Alcohol-Related Problems                    No. 99
⊕ http://www.cma.ca/canmed/policy/alcohole.htm

A Canadian perspective on alcohol and alcohol-related problems is presented by the Canadian Medical Association (CMA). Reasons for why the CMA regards alcohol abuse as a major concern in Canada and information about the CMA's recommendation that Canadians adopt a policy to reduce alcohol consumption are detailed.

### Dispelling Myths About Alcohol                    No. 100
⊕ http://www.cts.com/crash/habtsmrt

Habit Smart presents "Information Drives Change." Looks for details on cognitive therapy, codependency, a self-scoring alcohol checkup, and more. A list of related sites is included.

### Duke University: Alcohol and Health Page                    No. 101
⊕ http://h-devil-www.mc.duke.edu/h-devil/drugs/alcohol.htm

This Duke University site outlines the hazards of alcohol. Several charts on the effects of drinking, the relationship of alcohol to body weight and blood alcohol content are included in this text-only page. Short and long term effects of alcohol consumption are presented, including nutritional complications, liver diseases, gastrointestinal problems, hangovers, and the effects on blood glucose. Questions may be posed through the Healthy Devil Online homepage.

### National Clearinghouse for Alcohol and Drug Information                    No. 102
⊕ http://www.health.org

Prevention Online presents this site on alcohol and drugs, which includes a list of electronic publications. Easy-to-use icons link a visitor to the latest information and research, statistics, online forums, searchable databases, and other resources.

### National Organization of Fetal Alcohol Syndrome (NOFAS)                    No. 103
⊕ http://www.nofas.org/

This developing site from NOFAS defines Fetal Alcohol Syndrome (FAS) and presents FAS resources. Other topics include information on NOFAS, strategies for working with FAS children, and a NOFAS medical school curriculum.

## Making Your Own Connections

**Address/URL**

**Notes/Observations/
Site Description**

http://
_____
_____
_____
_____

http://
_____
_____
_____
_____

http://
_____
_____
_____
_____

http://
_____
_____
_____
_____

## Making Your Own Connections

| Address/URL | Notes/Observations/ Site Description |
|---|---|
| http:// | |
| http:// | |
| http:// | |
| http:// | |

A goal of nutrition education, whether it is taught in elementary or secondary school, college, worksite, or in the community, is to provide knowledge and skills for successful living in a changing world. Nutrition education is the process by which attitudes, environmental influences, beliefs, and understanding about food as it relates to optimal health leads to practices that are nutritionally sound, realistic, and consistent with individual needs and available food sources. Nutrition education can provide the knowledge to make informed food choices in supermarkets, vending machines, and restaurants. Consumers today are faced with a dizzying array of manufactured and restaurant food items.

Although food labels can help people make choices, many labels are hard to understand or are misleading. Many consumers are confused by the term "low fat." Some assume lowfat automatically means low calorie, which is not always the case. Another confusing term is "cholesterol free." Cholesterol is found only in animal products; all vegetable foods are naturally free of cholesterol. Unfortunately, some cholesterol-free foods are high in saturated fats, which elevate blood cholesterol. The cholesterol-free label implies the product is heart healthy, which is not always true.

Schools are an ideal place to teach nutrition. The topic can be integrated into other courses and into the school lunch program. For example, the federal government has recently launched a nutrition education initiative called "Team Nutrition" to help children make food choices for a healthy diet and to implement changes in the national school lunch program. (Source: "What's for Lunch," *Mothering*, January/February 1997.) Teachers have many nutrition education resources available for all grades. Many resources are developed by industry (e.g., the National Dairy Council); others are produced by nonprofit sources or by the government. From the Office of Analysis and Evaluation, Food and Consumer Service comes a study on nutrition education programs and activities available in public elementary and secondary schools. (Source: *Family Economics & Nutrition Review*, Volume 9, 1996.) Other sources include "Resources for Teachers." (Source: *Curriculum Review*, September 1996.) Integrating nutrition into other courses is an interesting way to present the material. Reading recipes and labels in math, and teaching digestion and absorption in science are only two ways to include nutrition in other disciplines. As the number of overweight children increases, it is more important than ever to provide nutrition education in the schools.

# Nutrition Education

 Why are the schools a good place to teach nutrition? • How can nutrition be integrated into other disciplines? • Why are food labels hard to understand or even misleading?

## ⬤WebLinks

**Healthy School Meals Training Materials Database**     No. 104

⬤ http://schoolmeals.nal.usda.gov:8001/resources/hsmdbase.html

This searchable database for school nutrition personnel includes educational materials produced by universities, associations, industry, and government agencies. Links lead to information on healthy school meals, training, and publications from the National Agricultural Library.

**Nutrition Education for Grades Preschool–6**     No. 105

⬤ http://www.nalusda.gov/fnic/pubs/bibs/edu/preschool.html

The Food and Information Service of the U. S. Department of Agriculture presents details about available materials and audiovisuals on nutrition education for preschool through grade 6. The extensive information provides lesson plans on healthy eating, resources for adults and access to nutrition software.

**Nutrition Education Materials from WIC**     No. 106

⬤ http: www.nal.usda.gov/fnic/

Presented by the Food and Nutrition Information Center of the U. S. Department of Agriculture, visitors can use keywords to search for desired topics. Nutrition guidelines, research briefs, and nutrition education material are included. Links to information about healthy school meals and the food pyramid are provided.

**Nutrition Expedition**     No. 107

⬤ http://www.fsci.umn.edu/nutrexp/

This series of games for teachers and students can serve as a resource for nutrition education for grades K–12. The site is maintained by the University of Minnesota.

## Making Your Own Connections

| Address/URL | Notes/Observations/<br>Site Description |
| --- | --- |

http://

_____

_____

_____

http://

_____

_____

_____

http://

_____

_____

_____

http://

_____

_____

_____

## Making Your Own Connections

| Address/URL | Notes/Observations/Site Description |
|---|---|
| http:// | |
| http:// | |
| http:// | |
| http:// | |

# Nutrition Journals Online 24

Journals are legitimate sources of information and research on nutrition and health issues. There are literally hundreds of journals related to these topics. In addition to journals, there are equally large numbers of magazines that address topics in health, nutrition, and dieting. Which is the best source for obtaining accurate and valid information? What is the difference between journals and magazines? Generally, journals, written mostly for and by professionals, are considered a more reliable source. Although a magazine such as *American Health* offers up-to-date information about nutrition and health topics, its articles are usually written for the general public. A journal will almost always have one or more authors who are health and/or nutrition professionals. Magazines may use staff journalists to write their articles. In addition, journal articles are almost always referenced. A reference list at the end of the article identifies all the sources cited in the body of the paper, which allows the reader to verify these sources. A magazine article usually has no citations appearing at the end. Furthermore, a magazine article may report on a study which appeared in a journal, but the journal article is the *original* source. Journal articles must also be reviewed by fellow scientists before they can be published; magazines generally do not undergo such screenings.

The field of nutrition derives data through scientific research. Scientists need to systematically conduct research investigations and cautiously interpret the findings before they can offer practical nutrition information. They then report their findings in respected scientific journals. Work must survive a screening review by an author's peers before it is accepted for publication. Using a nutrition journal that is peer-reviewed and referenced is a good way to ensure your information is valid.

The following is a list of respected nutrition journals:

*Nutrition Reviews* is a publication of the International Life Sciences Institute. It offers recent evidence on current topics and presents extensive bibliographies. It is available monthly from Springer-Verlag New York, 175 Fifth Avenue, New York, NY 10010.

*Nutrition Today* is a magazine for laypeople. It covers controversial issues and provides a forum for conflicting opinions. Bimonthly issues are available from Williams and Wilkins, 428 East Preston Street, Baltimore, MD 21202.

*Nutrition and the M.D.* is a monthly newsletter that provides current, practical information on nutrition for healthcare providers. The address is PM, 7100 Hayven Hurst Avenue, Suite 107, Van Nuys, CA 91406.

# Nutrition Journals Online

Many journals put their tables of contents, past articles, and some current articles on the Web. These journal articles can be viewed, though the entire journal does not appear online.

- For research projects, would you choose a journal or magazine?
- How can you tell if a magazine article is offering valid information?

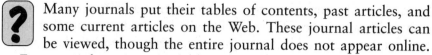

### American Journal of Clinical Nutrition                                  No. 108
🌐 http://www.faseb.org/ajcn/

This site is presented by the American Society for Clinical Nutrition, Inc. Visitors can view the contents of the current journal and access "New and Noteworthy" information. A link leads to "Cool Sites," which offers connections to other nutrition-related pages.

### British Journal of Nutrition                                            No. 109
🌐 http://www.cup.org/Journals/JNLSCAT/nut/nut.html

The *British Journal of Nutrition* is owned and published by the Massachusetts Medical Society. Information about the journal and a table of contents for each issue is available at the site (also available directly via E-mail). Look for a quiz and hot keys that lead to the journal, a homepage, or catalog.

### Journal of the American Dietetics Association                           No. 110
🌐 http://www.eatright.org/journaltoc.html

This site offers the table of contents for the current and previous issues of the *Journal of the American Dietetics Association*. Valid nutrition and dietetic practice information is presented. Hot keys allow visitors to search for dietitians, browse FAQs, read up-to-date information, and access other nutrition resources.

### Meducation-Journals                                                     No. 111
🌐 http://www.meducation.com/journal.html

Meducation provides medical education research journals on the World Wide Web. This site contains an alphabetical hyperlist of more than 80 medical, science, nutrition, and health journals. Abstracts and even full-text articles are available from many of the journals.

### New England Journal of Medicine                                         No. 112
🌐 http://www.nejm.org

This page offers a table of contents for each issue (also available directly via E-Mail), weekly journal reports on the results of important worldwide medical research, medline links, and search engines for further research. Although it is a medical journal, many of the articles are devoted to nutrition and diet. The site is maintained by the Massachusetts Medical Society, owner and publisher of the journal.

## Making Your Own Connections

Address/URL

Notes/Observations/
Site Description

http://
_____
_____
_____
_____

http://
_____
_____
_____
_____

http://
_____
_____
_____
_____

http://
_____
_____
_____
_____

# Nutrition Journals Online

## Making Your Own Connections

Address/URL

Notes/Observations/
Site Description

http://
_____
_____
_____
_____

http://
_____
_____
_____
_____

http://
_____
_____
_____
_____

http://
_____
_____
_____
_____

# Nutrition Through the Life Cycle 25

Throughout our lives, diet and nutrition can affect our health and wellbeing. Although most people are aware that during pregnancy, infancy, and childhood we need adequate protein, calcium, and iron, not everyone is aware that adults and seniors have important nutritional needs, too. A healthy diet, eaten throughout life, can have an impact on longevity and quality of life.

Humans have always attempted to prolong youth and life. The search goes on today. Scientists who study the process of aging have found that no specific diet or nutritional supplements will prolong life, but they have identified several links to nutrition. For instance, the lifestyle factors that can make a difference in aging are regular balanced meals, weight control, and regular physical activity. Unfortunately, although many elderly individuals have made positive dietary changes, a significant number do not get regular exercise. Lack of exercise is linked to decreased muscle and bone mass. A decline in muscle mass causes age-related decreases in strength, activity, and metabolic rate. A lowered metabolic rate reduces the need for calories. As a result, many elderly individuals need considerably fewer calories than when they were younger. But most older people do not significantly reduce their caloric intake as their exercise rates fall, leading to increased body fatness, especially in the abdominal area. Abdominal fat is linked to adult diabetes, which has been increasing steadily in the United States. (Source: "Nutrition, Exercise, and Healthy Aging," *Journal of the American Dietetics Association,* June 1997.)

Besides diabetes, Alzheimer's disease also affects as many as five percent of individuals by age 65 and 20 percent of those over age 80. (Source: "Progress Report on Alzheimer's Disease," *National Institutes of Aging,* NIH publication 94-3885, 1994.) Alzheimer's disease causes the brain to deteriorate abnormally, with death of brain cells occurring in areas of the brain that affect cognition and memory. Nutrition seems to be only weakly linked to Alzheimer's. Brain aluminum in people with the disease exceeds normal brain aluminum by 10 to 30 times. It is unclear, however, if the high brain aluminum is a result rather than the cause of Alzheimer's disease. The nutrition link to Alzheimer's is unclear, but nutrient deficiencies, particularly those that continue over many years, may contribute to the memory loss and impaired cognition that affect many older adults. These deficiencies are not thought to cause Alzheimer's, and they can be mostly reversed by a healthy diet. (Source: "Growing Older, Eating Better," *FDA Consumer,* March 1996.)

# Nutrition Through the Life Cycle

 Why do older people need fewer calories than their younger counterparts? • What is the relationship between diet and memory loss? • Can Alzheimer's disease be treated with diet?

## ●WebLinks

### Alzheimer's Association                                              No. 113
● http://www.alz.org

Visit the Alzheimer's Association's homepage to learn about the organization, the latest in the news, caregiver resources, public policy, and conferences and events. Links to related resources and research are provided.

### Children's Nutrition Research Center                                 No. 114
● http://www.bcm.tmc.edu/cnrc/

The Children's Nutrition Research Center at the Baylor College of Medicine is sponsored by the U.S. Department of Agriculture. This page offers a research overview, "Nutrition and Your Child" newsletter, the latest news, details on seminars, and links to related material. The page was honored as a Top 5% Web Site.

### Jean Mayer United States Department of Agriculture,
### Human Nutrition Research Center on Aging                             No. 115
● http://www.hnrc.tufts.edu

The Jean Mayer United States Department of Agriculture, Human Nutrition Research Center on Aging studies the effects of human nutrition on health. Links provided take visitors to an introduction of the center, research programs, human studies programs, and scientific publications.

### National Institutes of Aging                                        No. 116
● http://www.nih/gov/nia

Look for information on the National Institutes of Aging, research, funding, and training through links provided here. The latest news and related sites are also available.

# Nutrition Through the Life Cycle

## *Making Your Own Connections*

Address/URL

Notes/Observations/
Site Description

http://
_____

_____

_____

_____

http://
_____

_____

_____

_____

http://
_____

_____

_____

_____

http://
_____

_____

_____

_____

# Nutrition Through the Life Cycle

## Making Your Own Connections

| Address/URL | Notes/Observations/ Site Description |
|---|---|
| http:// | |
| http:// | |
| http:// | |
| http:// | |

# Pregnancy

A woman who is pregnant, or who may be at some time, needs to know that her nutrition today will be critical to the wellbeing of the child to come. The nutrition demands of pregnancy are outstanding because the growth of a new human being requires every known nutrient, and extra amounts of most of them.

To ensure they are nourishing themselves optimally for their infants-to-be, women need to start eating healthy before they are pregnant. In early pregnancy, significant development of the embryo depends on a woman's nutrition status prior to becoming pregnant. A maternal deficiency of the B vitamin folate has been linked to the development of a variety of birth defects, including spina bifida (spinal cord bulge through the back) and anencephaly (absence of a complete brain). These conditions cause paralysis, incontinence, hydrocephalus, and learning disabilities. It has been estimated that nearly half of all neural tube defects could have been prevented with adequate folate intake. Since about half of all pregnancies in the United States are unplanned, it would be prudent for all women to consume diets rich in folate. Food sources of this vitamin include leafy vegetables, fortified cereals, oranges, strawberries, cantaloupe, liver, and beans. (Source: "Folate and Neural Tube Defects," *Nutrition Reviews*, Volume 53, 1995.)

Although folate is essential during pre- and early pregnancy, what about other vitamins and minerals? Do pregnant women need supplements? In general, most pregnant women in the U. S. receive prescriptions for prenatal vitamins from their health providers, though, with the exception of iron supplements, these are not necessarily recommended by most scientific organizations. Taking prenatal vitamins along with a healthy diet can help ensure a healthy baby. Taking large doses of vitamins during pregnancy, however, has been related to some health concerns. Large doses of vitamin A from supplements has been linked to birth defects. (Source: "The Vitamin A Scare, The Beta Carotene Answer," *Let's Live*, January 1996.)

Other nutritional risk factors for pregnant women include alcohol consumption, not enough iron, inadequate protein, too many calories, and weight gain. Pregnancy is not a time to diet even if a woman is overweight at the beginning of the pregnancy. On average, a minimum 25–35 pound weight gain is recommended during the course of a full-term pregnancy. (Source: "Supplementation, Not Dieting," *Better Nutrition*, April 1996.) Ideally, this weight gain should include milk products, fruits and vegetables, whole grains, and lean protein foods.

# Pregnancy

**?** Why should women of childbearing age pay attention to diet even if they are not currently pregnant? • What nutrient can help to prevent neural tube defects? • Why do pregnant women especially need an adequate intake of fruits and vegetables?

## ⬤WebLinks

### American College of Obstetricians and Gynecologists          No. 117
 ⬤ http://www.acog.com/

The American College of Obstetricians and Gynecologists is an organization of women's health care physicians. The site offers member access, news releases, publications, a catalog, and information about the organization.

### Archives of Gynecology and Obstetrics          No. 118
 ⬤ http://link.springer.de/link/service/journals/00404/index.htm

This simple site provides information on, and the contents of, the journal, *Archives of Gynecology and Obstetrics*. Look for announcements posted from the journal.

### Mayo Clinic Health Oasis: Pregnancy & Child Health Resource Center No. 119
 ⬤ http://www.mayo.ivi.com/ivi/mayo/common/htm/pregpg.htm

Maintained by the Mayo Clinic, this user-friendly site features reference articles, a due date calculator, advice about sex during pregnancy, and parenting information. The opportunity to ask questions of clinic physicians and links to related sites benefit visitors.

### U.S. Food and Drug Administration, Center for Food Safety
### and Applied Nutrition: Information for Women Who Are Pregnant          No. 120
 ⬤ http://vm.cfsan.fda.gov/~dms/wh-preg.html

Links-only site offers sensible information from the Center for Food Safety and Applied Nutrition of the U.S. Food and Drug Administration. Topics include eating for two, folate and neural tube defects, vitamin A and birth defects, healthy eating during pregnancy, breastfeeding, and infant formula.

# Making Your Own Connections

Address/URL

Notes/Observations/
Site Description

http://
_____
_____
_____

http://
_____
_____
_____

http://
_____
_____
_____

http://
_____
_____
_____

## Making Your Own Connections

**Address/URL**

**Notes/Observations/
Site Description**

http://

_____

_____

_____

http://

_____

_____

_____

http://

_____

_____

_____

http://

_____

_____

_____

_____

# Professional Organizations 27

Most professionals have at least one organization that represents their field. These organizations provide member services, which may include credentialing, practice standards, information dissemination, job banks, career guidance, and continuing education programs. Professional organizations are usually made up of active and retired professionals in the field and sometimes students and interested laypersons. Numerous professional organizations exist in the nutrition field, including dietetic practice, clinical research, medical practices, eating disorders associations, and others. Examples of professional organizations include the American Dietetics Association, the American Society for Clinical Nutrition, the National Institute of Nutrition, The Nutrition Foundation, and the American Public Health Association. In addition to these professional groups, there are also organizations associated with specific diseases and illnesses. Examples of these organizations include The American Cancer Society, The American Health Association, The American Diabetes Association, and The American Anorexia and Bulimia Association.

How do professional organizations differ from trade associations? In general, trade associations are organizations associated with industry. For instance, the National Dairy Council (O'Hare International Center, 10255 West Higgins Road, Suite 900, Rosemond, IL 60018) is a trade association that promotes the use of dairy products. One means of this promotion has been the development and implementation of educational packages for grades K–12. The Dairy Council sells these packages to schools throughout the country. Although the information is valid, the underlying message is to use dairy products. Professional organizations do not sell or generally endorse specific products. They do endorse their profession.

For students and the general public, professional organizations are sources of reliable health and nutrition information, which is not related to specific products, such as meat or dairy foods. Many professional organizations also provide audiovisual materials, pamphlets, and journals. Organizations that provide these materials include American Institute of Nutrition (9650 Rockville Pike, Bethesda, MD 20814), Dietitians of Canada (480 University Avenue, Suite 604, Toronto, Ontario M5G 1V2, Canada), and the Nutrition Information Service (University of Alabama at Birmingham, Room 447 Webb Building, UAB Station, Birmingham, AL 35294).

# Professional Organizations

**?** Why would professional organizations often be the best source of valid nutrition materials? • Why might trade associations produce biased information? • Who becomes members of professional organizations?

## ⊘WebLinks

### American College of Clinical Nutrition     No. 121
⊘ http://www.faseb.org/ascn/

This site is maintained by the American College of Clinical Nutrition, a division of the American Society for Nutritional Sciences. It features hot keys that provide access to position papers, press releases on nutrition topics, and information on related nutrition organizations. Visitors may express comments through E-mail.

### American Dietetics Association     No. 122
⊘ http://www.eatright.org

The American Dietetics Association and its National Center of Nutrition and Dietetics promote optimal nutrition, health, and well being. This easy-to-navigate homepage presents FAQs about nutrition and dieting, nutrition and dieting resources, and career and member information. A nutrition survey, a tip of the day, and help in finding a dietitian are also available. Links connect to related sites.

### American Medical Association     No. 123
⊘ http://www.ama-assn.org

Lots of detail is provided in this user-friendly site. Look for information about advocacy, examine journals, review press releases, and read an overview of the organization. Links provide access to related topics.

### American Public Health Association     No. 124
⊘ http://www.apha.org

Public health resources, news, legislation and publications are accessed through links from the American Public Health Association page. The site has a public policy or political slant on health issues.

### The American Society of Parental and Enteral Nutrition (ASPEN)     No. 125
⊘ http://www.peakcom.com/clinnutr.org/

The American Society of Parental and Enteral Nutrition seeks to ensure that all patients receive optimal nutritional care. The site allows visitors to post questions or register for an audio teleconference on health topics. Look for nutrition standards and guidelines or read the current Clinical Dilemma Online. Links provide additional information on this and similar organizations.

### International Union of Nutritional Societies     No. 126
⊘ http://www.monash.edu.au/IUNS/index.htm

Lots of links throughout this Australian site offer access to global nutrition information. Learn about dietary guidelines, food facts, conferences, and visit the "link of the month."

## Making Your Own Connections

Address/URL

Notes/Observations/
Site Description

http://
_____
_____
_____

http://
_____
_____
_____

http://
_____
_____
_____

http://
_____
_____
_____

# Professional Organizations

## *Making Your Own Connections*

| Address/URL | Notes/Observations/ Site Description |
|---|---|
| http:// | |
| http:// | |
| http:// | |
| http:// | |

# Quackery/Nutritional Fraud  28

According to the U.S. Food and Drug Administration (FDA), two of the top ten health frauds in the United States are nutrition-related: weight loss and nutrition schemes. Consumers waste millions of dollars each year on nutritional fraud and quackery—unproven practices, supplements, or devices that claim to promote weight loss, weight gain, muscle growth, or health and vitality. The products include nutritional supplements, amino acid powders, and various weight reduction supplements. (Source: "Weight Loss Quackery," *National Council Against Health Fraud Newsletter,* July/August 1996.) Other unproven weight loss products are a variety of fiber pills, exercise devices, diet books, foot massagers, and an assortment of unsafe and often expensive products. Many overweight individuals want to believe that these materials will succeed after diets and exercise have failed. (Source: "Kenney Picks a Bone With The Zone," *NCAHF Newsletter,* December 1996.)

Some nutritional products are advertised as energy enhancers. "Super blue green algae," sold by over 200,000 independent distributors, promises that people who take these pills and powders will have increased vitality, less stress, relief from allergies, and appetite control. The advertising also claims that the product has an abundance of vitamins, minerals, and trace minerals. It costs $68 for two ounces. Could any of this be true? According to the *Tufts University Diet and Nutrition Letter* (July 1996), the product is basically pond scum that floats on brackish waters. Its only benefit is the money it makes for the independent distributors who sell it. It also contains fewer vitamins and minerals than a serving of broccoli. This product, for some reason, keeps growing in popularity. It currently has over 120 Web pages devoted to the aggressive marketing of these supplements.

In addition to blue green algae, other products such as bee pollen, spirolina, and various herbal diet compounds have been big sellers. Dr. Stephen Barrett, MD, who received the FDA Commissioner's Special Citation Award for fighting nutrition quackery, advises consumers to stay away from all supplements sold by independent distributors, people who market pills and capsules person-to-person. He examined the offerings of more than 50 companies whose nutrition products are sold that way and concluded that these items are expensive and often marketed with false claims as to their effectiveness.

Generally, if a diet book or product makes promises that sound too good to be true (eat your favorite foods and still lose weight), it probably is. Ignoring testimonials and keeping informed can help protect us from nutrition quacks.

# Quackery/Nutritional Fraud

**?** Why do so many people purchase unproven diet products? • How can you determine if a product will do what it promises? • Would you follow the advice of a non-professional working in a health food store?

## ●Web*Links*

### Center for Food Safety and Applied Nutrition: Protecting Yourself Against Health Fraud                    No. 127
● http://vm.cfsan.fda.gov/~dms/wh-fraud.html

The Center for Food Safety and Applied Nutrition of the U.S. Food and Drug Administration provides this key site. Links feature presentations of major health frauds and information from the Federal Trade Commission and the National Fraud Information Center.

### FDA Consumer Magazine                    No. 128
● http://www.fda.gov/fdac/796_toc.html

This magazine is published by the U.S. Food and Drug Administration (FDA). The modest site features consumer issues, updates, investigators' reports, and cases illustrating regulatory and administrative actions such as inspections, recalls, seizures, and court proceedings involving food and drugs. Visitors can link to back issues or the FDA's homepage as well as related subjects.

### Online Scams                    No. 129
● http://www.quackwatch.com/02ConsumerProtection/onscam.html

Maintained by Quackwatch, this site provides a text-only overview of fraud on the Internet and Web. Warning signs of questionable online advertising, tips to avoid fraud and a warning from the Federal Trade Commission are presented. Links and phone numbers to the National Fraud Information Center and the Federal Trade Commission are included.

### Quackwatch: Your Guide to Health Fraud, Quackery, and Intelligent Decisionmaking                    No. 130
● http://www.quackwatch.com

Learn to spot and avoid "Web quackery" with help from this site operated by Stephen Barrett, M.D. Numerous links lead to information on questionable products and services, general observations, publications for sale, and an overview of Quackwatch.

# Quackery/Nutritional Fraud

## Making Your Own Connections

Address/URL

Notes/Observations/
Site Description

http://

http://

http://

http://

# Quackery/Nutritional Fraud

## Making Your Own Connections

**Address/URL**

**Notes/Observations/
Site Description**

http://
_____
_____
_____
_____

http://
_____
_____
_____
_____

http://
_____
_____
_____
_____

http://
_____
_____
_____
_____

# Trade Associations 29

Many food manufacturers, growers, and producers have joined together to form trade associations. These groups represent, advertise, and promote their product(s). They include growers of fruits and vegetables (United Fresh Fruit and Vegetable Association, 727 North Washington Street, Alexandria, VA 22314; 800-336-3065); producers of rice (USA Rice Council, PO Box 740123, Houston, TX 77274), and food manufacturers (Beech-Nut, Checkerboard Square, 1B, St. Louis, MO 63164; 800-523-6633). Trade associations will often provide pamphlets, recipes, and other materials related to their products.

Other trade groups publish newsletters designed for health and nutrition professionals. The National Live Stock and Meat Board's Research and Nutrition Information Department publishes *Food & Nutrition News*, a newsletter highlighting nutritional aspects of meat and livestock. Published six times per year, it also includes "Nutrition Potpourri," short articles on similar topics. (Source: National Live Stock and Meat Board, 444 North Michigan Avenue, Chicago, IL 60611.) The United Soybean Board publishes *The Soy Connection*, a quarterly periodical written for nutrition professionals. It includes articles on the relationship of soy foods and health as well as recipes for incorporating soy products into a healthy diet. (Source: The United Soybean Board, Suite 110, Chesterfield, MO 63017.)

Food manufacturers also publish newsletters. Ross Products Division, a division of Abbott Laboratories, manufacturers of nutritional supplements and infant formulas, produces *Dietetic Currents*, a newsletter directed towards nutrition professionals. This periodical includes articles on timely nutrition topics as well as advertisements for Ross products. General Mills, the makers of breakfast cereals, publishes *Contemporary Nutrition*, also designed for nutrition professionals. Each publication contain articles written by eminent researchers, though it may also include ads and promotions for the company's products.

For the general public, trade associations are good sources of recipes, coupons, and creative ways to use the organization's products. Some trade associations also sponsor festivals such as the Buckwheat Festival in Penn Yan, New York and the Garlic Festival in Gilroy, California. Many of these promotions have parades, food booths, and other activities related to the product.

# Trade Associations

**?** What is the purpose of trade associations and who are their members? • What types of industries make up food trade associations? • What kinds of materials are available from trade associations? • Besides newsletters, what other activities are trade associations engaged in? • Are trade association materials valid? • What is the primary motive of trade associations?

## ●WebLinks

### Canadian Dairy Commission                                         No. 131
● http://www.agr.ca/cdc/cdc.html

The Canadian Dairy Commission presents this site in both English and French. It contains a search engine and list of related sites. Details include an overview and history of the commission, press releases, dairy data, industry policy, and programs and services.

### Chiquita Online                                                    No. 132
● http://www.chiquita.com

Banana facts and recipes, nutrition, and trivia can be found at this site. Included are histories of the banana and Chiquita Brands International, Inc., a list of company products, and a list of major markets. Links also supply information on licensing and job opportunities. The site is maintained by Chiquita Brands International, Inc.

### Florida Citrus Information                                         No. 133
● http://www.earth.net/output/florida/citrus/fl_citrus.html

Pell's Citrus and Nursery presents a brief history of citrus production in Florida, statistics on citrus growers, production data, nutritional information, and other citrus facts. Citrus fruits can be ordered through this site.

### Quaker Oats Company                                                No. 134
● http://www.quakeroats.com

Meet the chief executive officer, review the company and its history, and gain knowledge about the products of the Quaker Oats Company on this page sponsored by Quaker Oats. Press releases and information for investors are also provided.

### United Soybean Board                                               No. 135
● http://stratsoy.ag.uiuc.edu/~usb/welcome.html

This site offers information about the United Soybean Board, whose mission is to create an environment within which U.S. soybean producers can maximize profits and efficiency in production. Visitors can link to current and back issues of the *Soybean Sentinel*, the United Soybean Board newsletter, review the board's strategic plan, read annual reports, or learn about production and quality.

# Trade Associations

## Making Your Own Connections

Address/URL

Notes/Observations/
Site Description

http://
_____
_____
_____
_____

http://
_____
_____
_____
_____

http://
_____
_____
_____
_____

http://
_____
_____
_____
_____

## Making Your Own Connections

| Address/URL | Notes/Observations/ Site Description |
|---|---|
| http://_____ _____ _____ _____ | |
| http://_____ _____ _____ _____ | |
| http://_____ _____ _____ _____ | |
| http://_____ _____ _____ _____ | |

# Vegetarian Diets 30

An increasing number of people today are choosing to follow a vegetarian way of eating. There is more, however, to following a vegetarian diet than simply eating a greater amount of vegetables and eliminating meat. There are actually four major categories of vegetarian diets: vegans who avoid all animal flesh and all animal products (eggs and dairy); lacto vegetarians who include milk and milk products but avoid all other animal foods; lacto-ovovegetarians who use eggs and dairy but eliminate other animal products; and, according to Karen Inge, "new vegetarians" who eat a vegetable-based diet with only occasional inclusion of meat, poultry, and fish. (Source: "Vegetarianism," *Nutridate,* May 1996.) Why have an increasing number of people chosen to eliminate or reduce animal foods from their diet? Reasons include health, religion, or cultural or ethical concerns. Many individuals also believe that following a vegetarian diet will help them to lose weight. As a result, vegetarianism has become more popular.

Studies of vegetarians suggest that they often have significantly lower mortality rates from several chronic diseases, including cancer and cardiovascular disease than do meat eaters. This may be because diets of vegetarians tend to be lower in calories, cholesterol, and fat, especially saturated fat. Their diets are higher in fruits and vegetables, which lead to an increase in the intake of dietary fiber and antioxidant vitamins. (Source: "Vegetarian Diets," *Harvard Women's Health Watch,* January 1996.)

Although vegetarian diets can be a healthy alternative, due to the elimination of some food groups from the diet, vegetarians may be at risk for nutritional inadequacy. As the number of foods excluded increases so too does the risk of nutritional deficiency. As a result, individuals following a vegan diet would be at the greatest risk of not meeting their nutrient requirements, especially if the diet is poorly planned. (Source: Janette Marshall, "So You Want to Be a Vegetarian?" *Essentials,* April 1996.)

Vegetarian diets need to be carefully planned. The nutrients supplied by meat, fish, poultry, eggs, and milk need to be replaced by alternative sources. Simply removing the meat from the diet and eating more vegetables will not make a nutritionally complete vegetarian. Nutrients most at risk include protein, iron, zinc, calcium, and vitamin $B_{12}$ (for vegans). Good planning, however, can provide these nutrients for vegans and other vegetarians. Alternatives to animal foods such as soy milk, tofu, and veggie burgers can help vegetarians meet their nutritional needs. Dietary supplements are also an option.

# Vegetarian Diets

 Would you consider giving up animal products? • If so, how would you ensure that your diet met your nutritional needs? • How would you find vegetarian meals away from home?

## ●WebLinks

### Food and Drug Administration's Guide to Vegetarianism    No. 136
● http://fda.gov/opacom/catalog/vegdiet.html

The U.S. Food and Drug Administration presents a text-only document that reviews the advantages and disadvantages of a vegetarian diet. Links are supplied to connect visitors to dietary guidelines and supporting articles.

### North American Vegetarian Society    No. 137
● http://www.cyberveg.org/navs/

This site is maintained by the North American Vegetarian Society, an organization that promotes health, nutrition, and the environmental benefits of a meatless diet. Literature on vegetarianism and a list of affiliates are included. Available booklets and answers to FAQs can be assessed through supplied links.

### Soy and Human Health    No. 138
● http://spectre.ag.uiuc.edu/~stratsoy/soyhealth/

A joint effort of the University of Illinois and the Soybean Council, this site allows visitors to post questions for answers. Links connect to related Web sites, books and publications.

### Vegetarian Guide to Vegetarian Restaurants    No. 139
● http://catless.ncl.ac.uk/veg/Guide/index.html

The World Guide to Vegetarianism is a listing of vegetarian and vegetarian-friendly restaurants, stores, organizations, products, and services. Links allow visitors to restrict their searches to specific world regions. The site was honored as a Top 5% Web Site.

### The Vegetarian Resource Group    No. 140
● http://www.vrg.org

Vegetarianism in a nutshell. Review information on vegetarian journals, press releases, and updates at this interactive site. Vegetarian cookbooks, travel, and a game are also featured. Links available throughout.

## Making Your Own Connections

| Address/URL | Notes/Observations/ Site Description |
|---|---|
| http:// _____ _____ _____ _____ | |
| http:// _____ _____ _____ _____ | |
| http:// _____ _____ _____ _____ | |
| http:// _____ _____ _____ _____ | |

## Making Your Own Connections

**Address/URL**

**Notes/Observations/
Site Description**

http://
_____
_____
_____

http://
_____
_____
_____

http://
_____
_____
_____

http://
_____
_____
_____

# Vitamins, Minerals & Water ▪ 31

Millions of consumers regularly take vitamin and mineral preparations each day in hopes of staying healthy, treating disease, and increasing the energy. Do we need supplements or are we wasting large amounts of money on worthless products? For many people, nutritional supplements are an important part of their lives. Pregnant women, people with chronic diseases, and dieters all benefits from vitamin and mineral pills. Picky eaters, those who eat on the run, and anyone who is unable or unwilling to get the nutrients they need from diet also benefit. (Source: "The Great Vitamin Debate," *Good Housekeeping,* February 1996.) But could the rest of us benefit? Many healthy people are taking supplements to prevent disease even if they already eat a nutritious diet. For instance, vitamins C and E have been recommended to reduce the risk of death from coronary heart disease. A recent study suggested that, in post-menopausal women, the intake of vitamin E from food is associated with a reduced risk of death from heart attacks. (Source: "Dietary Antioxidants and Death from Coronary Heart Disease in Post Menopausal Women," *New England Journal of Medicine,* May 2, 1996.) It's not clear if supplements, as opposed to food, will offer the same benefit. It is also not certain if regular multiple vitamins offer any protection against chronic disease. A study conducted by the American Cancer Society and the Centers for Disease Control and Prevention found that regular multivitamin intake did not prevent heart trouble and stroke. (Source: "Multivitamins: Do They Measure Up?" *Health,* September 1996.)

While the debate continues, is there any harm in taking supplements? In large doses, some vitamin and mineral preparations are toxic, such as vitamins A and D, or may interfere with other nutrients. For instance, large amounts of calcium from supplements may reduce absorption of iron. (Source: "Ask the Experts: Calcium Intake," *Executive Health's Good Health Report,* March 1997.) There is always the risk that some people will assume that all their nutritional needs are being met if they take a supplement and not make an effort to eat a healthy diet. Supplements cannot take the place of food, which provides not only vitamins and minerals, but fiber, amino and fatty acids, and other important compounds. Supplements also provide large, concentrated amounts of a nutrient. Are humans able to absorb such large amounts? Researchers like Dr. Elizabeth Whalen believe that we are simply not able to utilize huge quantities of vitamins and minerals at a time. (Source: "Can You Beat the Odds," *Across the Board,* February 1996).

# Vitamins, Minerals & Water

 Which vitamins are toxic in large amounts? • What are the risks associated with using supplements? • Why do healthy people take vitamin and mineral pills?

## ⊕WebLinks

### Healthy Homepage—Vitamins        No. 141
⊕ http://www.vitamin.com/index.html

The homepage of Pharmavite Corporation offers news, press releases, and details about the company. The history and a tour of the facilities are available.

### Information about Dietary Supplements        No. 142
⊕ http://vm.cfsan.fda.gov/~dms/supplmnt.html

The Center for Food Safety and Applied Nutrition of the U.S. Food and Drug Administration (FDA) presents information about dietary supplements. This site contains links to several FDA warnings, published supplements, final regulation rulings, and proposed guidelines.

### Iron Not Linked to Heart Disease        No. 143
⊕ http://ificinfo.health.org/insight/iron.htm

This site is maintained by the International Food Information Council. The text-only document provides an update on the relationship between dietary iron and the risks of heart disease.

### Nutrition Supplements        No. 144
⊕ http://h-devil-www.mc.duke.edu/h-devil/nutrit/suppl.htm

Duke University provides a fact sheet on vitamin, mineral, and protein supplements. Although no links are included, questions may be posed through the Healthy Devil Online homepage.

### Refresher on Water        No. 145
⊕ http://ificinfo.health.org/insight/waterref.htm

A glossary and a search engine are featured at this text-only site. Maintained by the International Food Information Council, this fact sheet outlines water's lifeline, its risks, and the difference between hard and soft water.

### The Shake Out on Sodium        No. 146
⊕ http://ificinfo.health.org/insight/sodium.htm

Information on blood pressure and the role sodium plays in our bodies is provided by researcher Dr. David McCarron. This site, maintained by the International Food Information Council, is text-only and offers a glossary and a search engine.

## Making Your Own Connections

| Address/URL | Notes/Observations/ Site Description |
|---|---|
| http:// _____ _____ _____ _____ | |
| http:// _____ _____ _____ _____ | |
| http:// _____ _____ _____ _____ | |
| http:// _____ _____ _____ _____ | |

# Vitamins, Minerals & Water

## Making Your Own Connections

Address/URL

Notes/Observations/
Site Description

http://
_____
_____
_____

http://
_____
_____
_____

http://
_____
_____
_____

http://
_____
_____
_____

# Weight Loss Programs

## 32

There are numerous commercial as well as nonprofit weight loss programs. Some programs promote safe, healthy weight loss plans along with moderate exercise. Other programs offer dramatic, rapid weight loss while promising consumers they will be able to continue to eat their favorite foods. Some promote unproven or spurious weight-loss aids, including diuretics, spirulina, appetite suppressants, herbal ingredients, or amino acid supplements. Other programs misrepresent salespeople as "nutrition counselors" who are qualified to give advice in nutrition without a profit motive. Yet others collect large amounts of money at the start or require that clients sign contracts for costly, long-term programs. Many of these programs fail to inform clients about any risks related to weight loss. (Source: "The Rationalization of Obesity-Management Services," *American Journal of Clinical Nutrition,* Volume 62, 1995.)

To determine if a weight loss program is sound, the following questions should be asked: Will the program provide a reasonable number of calories or at least 1,200 per day? Will it provide enough variety of foods to avoid boredom? Diets that promote eating the same few foods each day, such as the bananas and skim milk diet, don't supply enough nutrients and staying on the program is unlikely. Does it offer a healthy balance of protein, fat, and carbohydrates? Does it promote a slow, steady weight loss as opposed to a quick loss? Losing weight quickly cannot only be dangerous, but usually the initial loss is largely fluid. The fluid weight is usually quickly regained when eating returns to a normal level.

People do not necessarily lose more weight if they participate in a group support program. Studies have shown that people who maintain their weight losses have several things in common. Those who develop social support systems seem to be the most successful. Another key factor is the ability to follow a written diet plan and keep records. Finally, those who are successful maintain regular physical activity. (Source: "A Classification System to Evaluate Weight Maintainers, Gainers, and Losers," *Journal of the American Dietetics Association,* May 1997.) A weight loss program can be a motivator for some people and can be beneficial as long as the diet plan promotes exercise and encourages healthy eating. People who join programs that only allow certain foods or meal replacements are not considering the long term goal—to not only lose weight, but to maintain the loss.

# Weight Loss Programs

**?** What are some of the considerations in choosing a weight loss program? • How can you evaluate the nutritional content of a weight loss program? • What do you need to consider to maintain long term goals for keeping weight off? • What resources, social and material, are helpful for people who want to lose weight? • What can you do to encourage weight loss besides dieting? • What criteria can be used to determine the validity of a weight loss program?

## ●WebLinks

### Choosing a Safe and Successful Weight-Loss Program                    No. 147
● http://www.niddk.nih.gov/Saf&Suc/Saf&Suc.html

This fact sheet from the National Institutes of Health describes how to choose a safe and effective weight loss program. No links are included, but general healthy diet guidelines are provided.

### Duke University Rice Diet Program                    No. 148
● http://www.ricediet.com/

Duke University's famous rice diet is outlined. Designed to help people lose weight, lower cholesterol, and lower blood pressure, the unique possibility of using the diet as treatment for diabetes, hypertension, obesity, or heart disease is discussed.

### First Place                    No. 149
● http://www.firstplace.org

Based on the American Diabetics Association meal plan, this site features recipes, FAQs, a newsletter, information on workshops, and a catalog.

### Nutri/System®                    No. 150
● http://www.nutrisystem.com/main.html

This site, maintained by Nutri/System, outlines the features and benefits of the plan. Does this plan meet the criteria outlined in Web Site No. 147?

### UCLA University Obesity Center                    No. 151
● http://www.ccon.com/uclarfo/

The Division of Clinical Nutrition at the UCLA School of Medicine offers a weight loss program that promises to be quick, safe, easy, and permanent.

### Weight Watchers                    No. 152
● http://www.weight-watchers.com/

This user-friendly site provides a global look at Weight Watchers. Visitors can access information about weight loss programs, wellness news and worldwide meetings and forums. Selecting one of the many national flag graphics provided will lead to information on Weight Watchers in that country.

# Weight Loss Programs

## Making Your Own Connections

Address/URL

Notes/Observations/
Site Description

http://
_____
_____
_____
_____

http://
_____
_____
_____
_____

http://
_____
_____
_____
_____

http://
_____
_____
_____
_____

## Making Your Own Connections

| Address/URL | Notes/Observations/ Site Description |
|---|---|
| http:// _____ _____ _____ _____ | |
| http:// _____ _____ _____ _____ | |
| http:// _____ _____ _____ _____ | |
| http:// _____ _____ _____ _____ | |

# Women's Nutrition

## 33

Nutrition is the key to women's health. It is at the forefront to the prevention and treatment of the most devastating diseases that affect women. Nutrition is one of the single biggest factors in the health and well being of a woman at any stage of her life. In premenopausal years, nutrition plays a key role in women's health during childbearing and lactation. In later years, women are prone to conditions such as breast cancer, heart disease, and osteoporosis, which have strong links to diet and nutrition. Nutrition research may make the difference in the prevention and treatment of these diseases.

Although the role of fat in breast cancer is inconclusive, women with dense breasts have an increased risk for the disease. Breast density is decreased with a low-fat diet. (Source: "Women in the New World Order," *Journal of the American Dietetics Association*, May 1997.) Other diet-breast cancer relationships have been demonstrated. A potentially major breakthrough is related to phytoestrogens, which are found in a wide variety of foods including soy products, whole grains, berries, and nuts. Phytoestrogens may reduce the risk of breast cancer by reducing the effects of the hormone estrogen. (Source: "Fiber, Phytochemicals, and Antioxidants: Their Relation to Breast Cancer," *Nutrition and the M.D.*, Volume 22, 1996.)

Heart disease, thought of as a man's disease, is the leading killer of women. An important strategy for reducing heart disease risk is weight control. Unfortunately, about one third of women in the U.S. are overweight, with the highest incidence among younger women, especially women of color. And it is not just obesity that increases the risk; it has more to do with where the fat is deposited. Abdominal fat, more common among older, post menopausal women, is associated with a higher risk of heart disease.

Osteoporosis is thought of as a women's disease. Men do get osteoporosis, but at a lower rate than women. One out of every two women will have an osteoporosis-related fracture in her lifetime. A diet rich in calcium along with exercise may reduce the risk. A low intake of sodium and protein may also help lessen the risk of developing osteoporosis.

Advances being made in nutrition and women's health hold great promise. Nutrition may prove to be the single most important contribution to disease prevention and treatment into the next century.

# Women's Nutrition

 Do you regularly get enough calcium in your diet? • Do you maintain ideal body weight? • What foods are rich sources of phytoestrogens?

## ●WebLinks

### Breast Cancer Net                                              No. 153
● http://www.breastcancer.net

Some newsrooms for keywords, access articles, and learn about treatments and support at this site from Breast Cancer Net. Links to related pages are included.

### Osteoporosis and Related Bone Diseases: National Resource Center   No. 154
● http://www.osteo.org/

The National Resource Center, which is supported by the National Institutes of Health, seeks to create awareness of osteoporosis and other bone diseases and the possibilities for therapy. Look for comprehensive links on what's new, osteoporosis and men, information about the center, and related pages.

### Women's Health Institute                                       No. 155
● http://www.womens-health.com

This interactive site promotes learning and growth. Information about cardio-vascular health with a personal heart health assessment, menopause issues, and mind body health is presented. Infertility, gynecological health, pregnancy factors, and more are also covered in this broad site. Links to an index, topic discussions, and additional resources are included.

### Women's Health Weekly                                          No. 156
● http://www.newsfile.com/x1w.htm

Updated weekly, this site provides the week's top stories along with women's health and nutrition updates. Links provide access to past issues.

### A Woman's Space                                                No. 157
● http://www.yoyoweb.com/wospace

This award-winning site provides links to a large variety of issues. Visitors can join discussion groups, browse through books and movies, learn more about health and nutrition, obtain recipes, or read more on work-related issues.

## Making Your Own Connections

| Address/URL | Notes/Observations/<br>Site Description |
|---|---|
| http:// | |
| http:// | |
| http:// | |
| http:// | |

## Making Your Own Connections

| Address/URL | Notes/Observations/ Site Description |
|---|---|
| http:// | |
| http:// | |
| http:// | |
| http:// | |

# World Hunger

## 34

Worldwide, as many as one in five adults and one in four children do not have enough calories and protein to maintain health and well-being. In the developing world, poverty and hunger are caused by a variety of conditions, including environmental changes, rapid population growth, politics, armed conflicts, education, cultural factors, and climactic changes. (Source: "The Politics of Hunger," *Earth Island Journal,* Spring 1997.) Environmental changes such as pollution of water, loss of topsoil, and the cutting forests ultimately affect hunger and poverty. These environmental changes also lead to climactic changes that can affect the availability of food.

Although the most obvious form of hunger is famine, millions of people suffer from less severe but chronic hunger. It is estimated that nearly 800 million people, mostly women and children, are chronically malnourished. An additional two billion women and children are deficient in vitamin A, iodine and iron resulting in anemia, blindness, goiter and related conditions. (Source: "Feeding the World," *Economist,* November 16, 1996.) Besides suffering from nutritional deficiencies, tens of thousands of people die from malnutrition every day. Most children who succumb to malnutrition actually die because their health has been affected by dehydration resulting from infections that cause diarrhea. Malnourished children are very susceptible to infections and diseases such as measles. Because of poverty, infection and malnutrition, the life expectancy in some developing nations averages less than 50 years compared to 75 years in developed countries. (Source: "When Relief Is Not Enough," *Christianity Today,* December 9, 1996.)

What solutions might reduce hunger and poverty in the world today? In developing nations, environmental degradation needs to be reversed: population growth lowered, better education provided, especially for girls and women, and services to the poor improved. Wealthier nations need to reduce their overuse of resources and lessen pollutants that are adding to global environmental changes.

Currently, many nations like the United States, Canada, and several western European countries have well-developed food aid programs to help the needy overseas. Various hunger relief organizations provide agricultural, nutrition, and health education, food donations, and medical supplies to developing countries. For famines and true food shortages that cause large numbers of people to starve, food aid has, in the short term, kept many from dying.

# World Hunger

**?** What are the causes of world hunger? • What percentage of adults in the world today don't have enough nutrients and calories to maintain health? How many children? • What recent environmental changes can impact world hunger? • What nutrients are most often deficient worldwide? • While the most severe form of hunger is famine, what are the dangers of chronic hunger or chronic malnutrition? • What solutions can help?

## ●WebLinks

### International Network of Food Data Systems (INFOODS)   No. 158
● http://www.crop.cri.nz/foodinfo/infoods/infoods.htm

The goal of INFOODS, which was created by the International Food Data Systems Project at the United Nations University Food and Nutrition Programme in New Zealand, is to improve data on the nutrient composition of foods from all parts of the world. This site includes an introduction to the agency and links leading to information on a training course and available materials such as publications, a newsletter, a directory, and software.

### International Service Agencies (ISA)   No. 159
● http://www.charity.org/

ISA's homepage provides links to a multitude of hunger relief agencies including Opportunity International, Educational Concerns for Hunger Organization, and American World Service. Visitors can find out about the program and support opportunities of these charity groups or contact them through E-mail.

### World Health Organization   No. 160
● http://www.who.ch/

Review a list of major programs and a world health report at this site presented by the World Health Organization. Lots of links and a search engine provide access to newsletters, directories, libraries, and events. Information for travelers and a list of regional offices are included. The site was honored as a Top 5% Web Site.

### World Neighbors Home Page   No. 161
● http://www.wn.org/index06.htm

This homepage presents an overview of World Neighbors, a nonprofit organization whose goal is to eliminate hunger, disease, and poverty in developing nations. An array of hot keys take visitors to a list of ongoing projects, news of recent partnerships, FAQs, and available publications. Related international development sites are also linked.

## Making Your Own Connections

| Address/URL | Notes/Observations/ Site Description |
|---|---|
| http:// | |
| http:// | |
| http:// | |
| http:// | |

## Making Your Own Connections

**Address/URL**

**Notes/Observations/
Site Description**

http://
_____
_____
_____
_____

http://
_____
_____
_____
_____

http://
_____
_____
_____
_____

http://
_____
_____
_____
_____

# How to Read the New Food Labels

**Serving Size**
Is your serving the same size as the one on the label? If you eat double the serving size listed, you need to double the nutrient and calorie values. If you eat one-half the serving size shown here, cut the nutrient and calorie values in half.

**Calories**
Are you overweight? Cut back a little on calories! Look here to see how a serving of the food adds to your daily total. A 5'4", 138-lb. active woman needs about 2,200 calories each day. A 5'10", 174-lb. active man needs about 2,900. How about you?

**Total Carbohydrate**
When you cut down on fat, you can eat more carbohydrates. Carbohydrates are in foods like bread, potatoes, fruits and vegetables. Choose these often! They give you more nutrients than **sugars** like soda pop and candy.

**Dietary Fiber**
Grandmother called it "roughage," but her advice to eat more is still up-to-date! That goes for both soluble and insoluble kinds of dietary fiber. Fruits, vegetables, whole-grain foods, beans and peas are all good sources and can help reduce the risk of heart disease and cancer.

**Protein**
Most Americans get more protein than they need. Where there is animal protein, there is also fat and cholesterol. Eat small servings of lean meat, fish and poultry. Use skim or low-fat milk, yogurt and cheese. Try vegetable proteins like beans, grains and cereals.

**Vitamins & Minerals**
Your goal here is 100% of each for the day. Don't count on one food to do it all. Let a combination of foods add up to a winning score.

## Nutrition Facts

Serving Size ½ cup (114g)
Servings Per Container 4

**Amount Per Serving**

**Calories** 90      Calories from Fat 30

**% Daily Value***

| | |
|---|---|
| **Total Fat** 3g | **5%** |
| Saturated Fat 0g | **0%** |
| **Cholesterol** 0mg | **0%** |
| **Sodium** 300mg | **13%** |
| **Total Carbohydrate** 13g | **4%** |
| Dietary Fiber 3g | **12%** |
| Sugars 3g | |
| **Protein** 3g | |

| | | | | |
|---|---|---|---|---|
| Vitamin A | 80% | • | Vitamin C | 60% |
| Calcium | 4% | • | Iron | 4% |

*Percent Daily Values are based on a 2000 calorie diet. Your daily values may be higher or lower depending on your calorie needs:

| | | Calories | 2000 | 2500 |
|---|---|---|---|---|
| Total Fat | Less than | | 65g | 80g |
| Sat Fat | Less than | | 20g | 25g |
| Cholesterol | Less than | | 300mg | 300mg |
| Sodium | Less than | | 2400mg | 2400mg |
| Total Carbohydrate | | | 300g | 375g |
| Fiber | | | 25g | 30g |

Calories per gram:
Fat 9  •  Carbohydrates  4  •  Protein  4

*More nutrients may be listed on some labels.*

g = grams (About 28 g = 1 ounce)
mg = milligrams (1,000 mg = 1 g)

**Total Fat**
Aim low: Most people need to cut back on fat! Too much fat may contribute to heart disease and cancer. Try to limit your **calories from fat.** For a healthy heart, choose foods with a big difference between the total number of calories and the number of calories from fat.

**Saturated Fat**
A new kind of fat? No — saturated fat is part of the total fat in food. It is listed separately because it's the key player in raising blood cholesterol and your risk of heart disease. Eat less!

**Cholesterol**
Too much cholesterol — a second cousin to fat — can lead to heart disease. Challenge yourself to eat less than 300 mg each day.

**Sodium**
You call it "salt," the label calls it "sodium." Either way, it may add up to high blood pressure in some people. So, keep your sodium intake low — 2,400 to 3,000 mg or less each day.*

* The AHA recommends no more than 3,000 mg sodium per day for healthy adults.

**Daily Value**
Feel like you're drowning in numbers? Let the Daily Value be your guide. Daily Values are listed for people who eat 2,000 or 2,500 calories each day. If you eat more, your personal daily value may be higher than what's listed on the label. If you eat less, your personal daily value may be lower.

For fat, saturated fat, cholesterol and sodium, choose foods with a low **% Daily Value.** For total carbohydrate, dietary fiber, vitamins and minerals, your daily value goal is to reach 100% of each.

# Appendix A

## You Can Rely on the New Label

Rest assured, when you see key words and health claims on product labels, they mean what they say as defined by the government. For example:

| Key Words | What They Mean |
|---|---|
| **Fat Free** | Less than 0.5 gram of fat per serving |
| **Low Fat** | 3 grams of fat (or less) per serving |
| **Lean** | Less than 10 grams of fat, 4 grams of saturated fat and 95 milligrams of cholesterol per serving |
| **Light (Lite)** | 1/3 less calories or no more than 1/2 the fat of the higher-calorie, higher-fat version; or no more than 1/2 the sodium of the higher-sodium version |
| **Cholesterol Free** | Less than 2 milligrams of cholesterol and 2 grams (or less) of saturated fat per serving |

| To Make Health Claims | The Food Must Be . . . About . . . |
|---|---|
| Heart Disease and Fats | Low in fat, saturated fat and cholesterol |
| Blood Pressure and Sodium | Low in sodium |
| Heart Disease and Fruits, Vegetables and Grain Products | A fruit, vegetable or grain product low in fat, saturated fat and cholesterol, that contains at least 0.6 gram soluble fiber, without fortification, per serving |

*Other claims may appear on some labels.*

# Citing a Web Site

Although a standard has not yet been developed for referencing on-line information, guidelines are in progress. The *MLA Handbook* and the *Publication Manual for the American Psychological Association* don't have full guidelines in their fourth editions, though electronic references can credit the author and enable readers to access the material. Many legitimate sources and references are on the Web, but some sites are advertisements and others have questionable validity.

Before citing from the World Wide Web (WWW), the following questions should be considered: Will the data be available to the reader or will the site quickly disappear? Is the data widely accessible or available only on a limited basis, e.g., a campus local network? In general, if both print and electronic forms of material are the same, the print form is preferred, though this may change as electronic forms become more available to researchers and libraries.

Electronic correspondence including E-mail, conversations via electronic discussion groups, and bulletin boards are cited as "personal communication" in the text according to the American Psychological Association. World Wide Web data files are cited in the text as author and date or, if no author is available, by the title of the file or home page. In the reference list, Web sites are cited by title of the data file, year, month, day, title of browser, address. An example is

"Prevention Primer" (1996, July 17.) National Clearinghouse for Alcohol and Drug Information. World Wide Web: http://www.health.org.

*Important note:* Before citing anything from the Internet and/or World Wide Web, be aware that much of what you may find, particularly related to nutrition, dieting and supplements, may not be valid. A recent study conducted by Davison and Guan found that, after accessing 167 nutrition-related documents, 45 percent of these provided information that was not consistent with one or more of established dietary guidelines and included advertisements recommending supplements, herbal remedies, weight-loss products, and specific diets. Internet resources continue to expand rapidly and nutrition professionals and students need to develop strategies to address inconsistent or questionable dietary information available through this technology. (Source: "The Quality of Dietary Information on the World Wide Web," *Journal of the Canadian Dietetics Association,* Winter 1996.)

# Appendix B

For further information on citing from the Web, see the following:

## In Print

American Psychological Association. (1995.) *Publication Manual of the American Psychological Association, 4th ed.* Washington DC: American Psychological Association.

Gibaldi, J. (1995.) *Handbook for writers of research papers 4th ed.* NY: Modern Language Association of America.

## Online

### MLA on the Web
✪ http://www.mla.org/

This is the site of the Modern Language Association. Here you will find guidelines on MLA documentation style. Click on *Citing Sources from the World Wide Web* and you will reach an easy-to-understand explanation on how to cite sources from the Web. A must-visit site. Text only, no links, but clear and authoritative examples provided.

### Classroom Connect: How to Cite Internet Resources
✪ http://www.classroom.net/classroom/CitingNetResources.html

Although written for K–12 educators, this site offers a good, clear "how-to" guide for referencing online sources in bibliographies. Some links to other sites.

### How to Cite Information from the Internet and the World Wide Web
✪ http://www.apa.org/journals/webref.htm

This brief page from the American Psychological Association explains the APA's recommendations for citing Web materials. Text only, no links.

## Your Personal Address Book

| Address/URL | Notes/Observations/<br>Site Description |
|---|---|

http://_____

_____

_____

_____

http://_____

_____

_____

_____

http://_____

_____

_____

_____

http://_____

_____

_____

_____

# Appendix C

## *Your Personal Address Book*

Address/URL

Notes/Observations/
Site Description

http://
_____
_____
_____
_____

http://
_____
_____
_____
_____

http://
_____
_____
_____
_____

http://
_____
_____
_____
_____

## Your Personal Address Book

| Address/URL | Notes/Observations/ Site Description |
|---|---|
| http:// | |
| http:// | |
| http:// | |
| http:// | |

# Appendix C

## *Your Personal Address Book*

Address/URL

Notes/Observations/
Site Description

http://

_____

_____

_____

http://

_____

_____

_____

http://

_____

_____

_____

http://

_____

_____

_____

# JumpStart Web Site Evaluation Form

Student Name _____

Date _____ Soc. Sec. # or Student I.D. # _____

Course Name & Number _____

Instructor Name _____

Web Site Name: _____

Site Number (if applicable) _____

Site Address/URL _____

**Briefly describe your online experience.** Were you able to access the site?

**Identify the Source / Who runs site.** Who is the person or what is the organization behind the site?

**Is the site links-intensive or content-intensive?** Or is it a combination of text and links to other sites?

**Provide a brief overview of site.** What resources and subjects or types of material are covered?

# Appendix D

How would you rate the quality of content? Was the information useful to you? If yes, how so? If not, why not?

How would you rate the quality of the site's graphics and its navigability/ease-of-use?

When was the site last updated?

What does this site offer compared to other sources of information used in this course?

# Let Us Hear From You

*JumpStart with WebLinks: A Guidebook for Nutrition, 98/99*

## Tell Us About Yourself

Name _____ Date _____

Are you a professor_____Are you a student _____

Your school name _____

Your Department_____

Address _____

City_____ State _____ Zip_____

Phone (Office): _____

E-mail:_____

Course number and title you used *JumpStart* for_____

Other texts/materials used for the course with *JumpStart*_____

_____

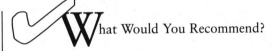 ## What Would You Recommend?

1. Are there any Web sites you feel should be deleted in the next edition of *JumpStart with WebLinks*? Please identify those sites by number and name and explain why.

2. Are there any Web sites that you think should be included in the next edition. Please provide the URLs (site addresses) and a brief description.

# ✄ Let Us Hear From You

### *JumpStart with WebLinks: A Guidebook for Nutrition, 98/99*

3. Are there topics that you would like to see dropped from *JumpStart* for the next edition?

4. Are there other topics that you would like to see included in the next edition?

5. Any other recommendations or advice?

May we quote you? _____

## Your thoughts are important to us!

## Tear out this page with your responses and mail it today!

Morton Publishing Company
925 W. Kenyon Ave., Unit 12
Englewood, CO  80110

Attn: *JumpStart with WebLinks*

# Index of WWW Sites with Page Number

# Index of WWW Sites with Page Number